REMEDIATING CHILDREN'S LANGUAGE

REMEDIATING CHILDREN'S LANGUAGE

BEHAVIOURAL AND NATURALISTIC APPROACHES

edited by
Dave J. Müller

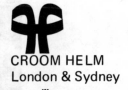

CROOM HELM
London & Sydney

COLLEGE-HILL PRESS, INC
San Diego, CA 92105

© 1984 Dave J. Müller
Croom Helm Ltd, Provident House, Burrell Row,
Beckenham, Kent BR3 1AT
Croom Helm Australia Pty Ltd, First Floor,
139 King Street, Sydney, NSW 2001, Australia

British Library Cataloguing in Publication Data

Remediating children's language.
   1. Children – Language
   2. Language disorders in children
   3. Remedial teaching
   I. Müller, David J.
   371.91'4   LB1139.L3

ISBN 0-7099-1766-X

College-Hill Press, Inc,
4284 41st Street
San Diego, CA 92105

Library of Congress Cataloging in Publication Data
Main entry under title:

Remediating children's language.

   Bibliography: p.
   Includes index.
   Contents: Introductory perspectives. Functional
analysis of verbal behavior / Derek E. Blackman–
Behavioural approaches to treating language disorders /
Donald E. Mowrer–Recent developments in pragmatics /
James McLean and Lee K. Snyder-McLean–[etc.]
   1. Language disorders in children–Patients–Rehabilitation.
2. Operant conditioning. 3. Reinforcement
(Psychology) I. Muller, Dave J.
RJ496.L35R46 1984   618.92'85506   84-7810
ISBN 0-933014-47-3

Printed and bound in Great Britain

CONTENTS

FIGURES

TABLES

To Vik

PREFACE

The idea for this book arose whilst I was involved with two colleagues in writing a textbook on language assessment (Müller, D.J., Munro, S., and Code, C. 1981, *Language Assessment for Remediation*, Croom Helm, London). In that book we included two brief chapters, one on the application of behaviourist techniques, the other on naturalistic considerations. It seemed to me at the time that these two areas were of extreme importance and that their significance was often overlooked in designing programmes to remediate children's language.

After finishing the first book I set about putting together the present text and soon came to the conclusion that it would need to be an edited volume if it were to reflect current research and practice in this field. Consequently, I selected the themes I thought to be of primary importance. These were a 'post-Chomskian' discussion of the theoretical basis for language remediation, some clear therapeutic guidelines on how to put theory into practice, and some critical viewpoints on which to base future research and clinical practice. My own view is that the contributors have done an excellent job for me in bringing out these perspectives and in producing material which is clearly of clinical relevance.

The book is intended for those with a professional interest in remediating children's language. It is aimed in particular at speech-language clinicians and pathologists, or speech therapists, but is likely also to be of relevance to teachers, and educational and clinical psychologists. The book has been edited with students of these professions in mind, but is at a sufficient level of sophistication to interest practitioners in the field. I hope it serves its main aim in demonstrating that behavioural techniques still have a significant part to play in children's language remediation, especially when linked to the child's natural environment.

I would like to thank my colleagues Pam Harris and Siân Munro for their careful reading of some of the chapters, Julia Hawkins for her administrative support and Lynne Conway for her typing. Finally, I would like to thank Vik, to whom this volume is dedicated, for her constant interest in my work.

Dave J. Müller

SECTION I: INTRODUCTORY PERSPECTIVES

The chapters in this section are aimed at re-establishing a clear theoretical and empirical rationale for using behavioural and naturalistic approaches when remediating children's language. Since the advent of 'Chomskian' linguistics, the notions that certain aspects of language might be learned and that intervention from an environmental perspective is to some extent behavioural, have become 'unfashionable'. It has become relatively easy to reject behavioural techniques on the grounds that language in its broadest sense could not be learned through a series of stimulus-response connections. This seems to have led to the assumption that behavioural principles are therefore inappropriate in a remediative context.

However, at the same time that behavioural principles have been rejected there has been an increasing awareness of the role of adults, and in particular mothers, in children's acquisition of language skills. These naturalistic considerations have emphasised the importance of behavioural techniques such as the use of reinforcement and prompting, without making explicit the theoretical basis for these principles. The heavy emphasis on 'innateness' and on non-empirical concepts such as 'deep structure' and 'competence', appear to have induced a reluctance to interpret recent studies on child language from a behavioural perspective. Yet, at the same time clinicians have been stressing the importance of working in the child's natural environment in order to foster language skills, implicitly through the use of behavioural techniques. It appears that clinicians in practice utilise behavioural techniques in naturalistic settings but feel unable to reject incompatible theoretical perspectives such as those offered by Chomsky. Consequently, insufficient consideration has been given to establishing a clear rationale for what clinicians actually do in practice, a concern shared by all the contributors to this section.

In the opening chapter, Blackman discusses Skinner's functional approach to verbal behaviour in the light of Chomsky's rather premature dismissal of this perspective. The potential value for language remediation of the experimental principles of operant conditioning are given careful consideration. Blackman argues that Skinner's analysis makes it possible to investigate empirically the concept of 'meaning' and this is reflected in the recent emphasis on pragmatics. It is made

1

clear that although functional analyses cannot entirely explain the acquisition and development of human language, it is possible to develop a system in which it can in principle be understood in terms of functional relationships between behaviour and environmental events. This approach is shown to provide a clear framework for the study of all aspects of language remediation.

In the next chapter Mowrer presents a detailed exposition of the principles of behaviourism and in an extensive literature review illustrates their use in modifying language. He shows the way in which language can be taught through altering the environmental input to evoke responses which can be shaped and maintained using selected schedules of reinforcement. Mowrer notes that the period between 1965 and 1975 marked the high point in the development of behavioural approaches and that since then there has been a steady decline, influenced he believes by the increased emphasis on linguistics and in particular generative grammar. He suggests that many of the behavioural approaches introduced into the classroom have been more innovative and imaginative than those designed to teach language skills to children and might profitably be adopted. This chapter goes some way to informing the reader of the range of behavioural techniques available and how they have been, and can be, used in clinical practice.

McLean and Snyder-McLean in the last chapter in this section illustrate the importance of utilising selected techniques in the context of the child's 'natural' environment. The authors discuss the remediative implications of recent developments in the study of pragmatics, which emphasises the use of language as a social tool. It is argued that the perspectives derived from theories and research in pragmatics direct clinicians to forms of intervention that have rarely been included in remediation. The key point is that language is seen as a way of influencing people and therefore children should be given the right and the ability to do this. This emphasis on the communicative and social functions of language is a predominant theme in the remainder of the chapters in this volume and is characteristic of the interface between behavioural and naturalistic approaches.

1 FUNCTIONAL ANALYSIS OF VERBAL BEHAVIOUR: A FOUNDATION FOR BEHAVIOURAL APPROACHES TO LANGUAGE REMEDIATION

Derek E. Blackman

'Relatively late in its history, the human species underwent a remarkable change: its vocal musculature came under operant control . . . Language was born, and with it many important characteristics of human behavior for which a host of mentalistic explanations have been invented' (Skinner, 1974, p. 88).

B.F. Skinner's own analysis of language and verbal behaviour appeared in its most extended form over a quarter of a century ago in the book which he developed from the William James lectures previously given at Harvard University (Skinner, 1957). In his book, Skinner provided a searching and essentially psychological analysis of speech and language which remains distinctive today. He addressed the challenge of understanding the diversity and complexity of our verbal behaviour by extrapolating in an adventurous and even daring way the principles which had been identified in laboratory studies of conditioned behaviour in animals. Skinner's theoretical bravado has not commanded wide support, however. Indeed in a historical context his book seems to have served rather as the basis for a polemical attack by Chomsky (1959) which provided the clarion call for the very different approaches to human language which largely characterise contemporary psycholinguistics. In general psycholinguists emphasise the uniqueness of human language and focus their studies on the structural characteristics of languages and of speech. This approach is sharply divergent from Skinner's programme, which is based on functional analyses of behaviour.

In this chapter an attempt is made to provide a sympathetic introduction to Skinner's functional account of verbal behaviour for readers who may not have encountered it or who may even have been encouraged to dismiss it peremptorily. Such a rehabilitative exercise is judged to be of value here not simply in historic or academic terms. Skinner's theory of language is an integral part of his approach to psychology as a whole. Through his research and writing Skinner has provided a coherent and unique system which embraces broad theoretical issues concerning the nature of language and yet also includes specific experimental principles which may be used, in the form of operant conditioning, for the more practical purposes of language remediation. The quotation with which this chapter opens illustrates this breadth of scope through its allusions to the appropriate explanation of language in general and to the control of the vocal musculature in particular.

Functional Analyses of Behaviour

In this section functional analyses of behaviour are introduced as a general explanatory system within psychology. In order to do this, some simple examples of experiments in the animal laboratory are briefly discussed, and the reader's indulgence should perhaps be craved here for this apparent diversion. It is important to emphasise at the outset that this foray into comparative psychology should not be taken to imply that human language is no more than a complicated version of rats' lever-pressing for reward in conditioning experiments, or indeed that rats are simplified, if 'furrier', versions of people. Some general explanatory *principles* which emerge clearly from experimental studies of animal behaviour, however, will subsequently be used in this chapter to address the mysteries and special richness of human language.

The animal experiments of relevance here are those described as operant conditioning. In a typical study a hungry rat is offered the opportunity to press a lever and thereby obtain a small pellet of food. It comes as no surprise to discover that in a well-conducted experiment the rat will press the lever repeatedly in this situation. As an increment of knowledge, this discovery is indeed of very limited impact. However, the *relationship* between the behaviour and its consequence provides the first component of a functional analysis of behaviour. If the delivery of food after a lever-press has an effect on the frequency with which the behaviour occurs, then a functional relationship between the two has been identified empirically. To characterise such a functional relationship, the consequence is then defined as a reinforcer and the behaviour as an operant response. If a consequence of behaviour serves to reduce the frequency of that behaviour the event can be termed a punisher. Punishers can therefore be defined, like reinforcers, in terms of their effects on an operant response. The terms operant response, reinforcer and punisher are properly used only if an appropriate functional relationship between the behaviour and its consequence has been identified. Thus in the experimental example the rat's lever-pressing is an operant response because it serves the function of producing a consequence, and that consequence is a reinforcer because it serves the function of maintaining the frequency of the behaviour. Note that the terms reinforcer and punisher are defined in these functional terms only, and there is no suggestion or supposition that they have any intrinsic pleasant or unpleasant qualities.

We have here a way of looking at behaviour, expressed in terms of its relationship with functionally significant consequences. This way of looking can be adopted to offer one account of behaviour which can sometimes be quite useful. For example, if we are asked why a rat is pressing a lever, one explanation of the behaviour might be in terms of its reinforcing consequences. Of course other explanations are by no means ruled out by such an analysis. An alternative account might be, for example, that the behaviour occurs because the rat is hungry, wants food, and has learned how to get it. The functional account, however, has the advantage of alerting us to a relationship between two observable events (behaviour and consequence) which has functional significance.

Experiments in operant conditioning have in fact extended our knowledge of how reinforcers can exert effects on behaviour even if they are related to the behaviour only occasionally. If reinforcers are delivered according to some schedule determined by the experimenter, the pattern and frequency of the operant responding will come to reflect that schedule. For example, when food is presented only after every twentieth lever-press a rat will come to press its lever at very high overall rates. On the other hand, if food becomes available for a lever-press only after a specified period of time has elapsed, then the operant responding will occur at much lower overall rates. Operant conditioning experiments have investigated the effects of many different schedules of intermittent reinforcement, thereby extending our ability to analyse different patterns of behaviour in functional terms.

We may now consider a second form of functional relationship which may develop between behaviour and environmental events, that termed discriminative control of behaviour. This too can be illustrated by a simple example. If an operant response is followed by a reinforcer only when some other feature of the environment is present (such as a light), then the operant responding will come to occur only when that feature is present and will not occur when it is absent. For example, if a light differentially accompanies periods when a schedule of reinforcement is in operation, then the rat will emit the typical pattern of operant responding with that schedule only when the light is present. In this case the light is termed a discriminative stimulus, again defined in terms of its functional relationship to behaviour. Discriminative stimuli are defined in terms of their function in setting the occasion for an operant response to occur (because of a schedule of reinforcement which is then in operation).

Operant conditioning experiments, then, provide experimental support for functional analyses of behaviour which direct our attention to the relationships between behaviour and events in the environment, discriminative stimuli and reinforcers or punishers. These functional analyses can be said to provide one coherent account of behaviour. The subtlety of the relationships which may develop between discriminative stimuli and behaviour and between behaviour and reinforcers or punishers may be such that a functional account provides a useful explanation of why the behaviour occurs, and thereby helps us to understand the behaviour better. The essential characteristic of this approach is that explanations of behaviour are couched in terms of the relationships between that behaviour and observable environmental events. Thus behaviour is in general conceptualised as a function of environmental conditions.

The literature of operant conditioning is extensive, revealing the power and subtlety of functional relationships between behaviour and environmental events in experimental conditions (see Blackman, 1974; Davey, 1981). However, it is the *principle* of functional analysis which provides the focus of the present discussion. It is the main thesis of contemporary behaviourists such as Skinner that the explanatory power of functional analyses of behaviour has often not been sufficiently recognised. Thus we tend not to favour explanations of behaviour expressed in these functional terms, preferring instead explanations in other terms, such as those related to underlying physiological or cognitive processes. This is particularly the case when we try to account for the behaviour of humans. Yet functional analyses of human behaviour in terms of discriminative stimuli and reinforcers or punishers can be both useful and powerful. Furthermore they are often the only explanations which are open to some form of empirical test and which therefore offer some promise as a satisfactory scientific account of human behaviour.

Functional accounts of human behaviour encourage us to analyse our own patterns of behaviour in terms of their relationships with antecedent and consequent events in the world around us. Such events are often provided by the people with whom we interact in social discourse. Teachers, for example, set out deliberately to change the behaviour of their pupils by selectively relating such things at their disposal as course grades or their own approval to behavioural changes in a desired direction ('learning'). The classroom provides the situation (discriminative stimulus) in which this selective reinforcement may occur. In a functional sense, then, certain patterns of behaviour on the part of pupils occur because of the discriminative properties of the learning situation and because of the reinforcement related to this behaviour in that situation. Thus learning is a function of the conditions provided by the teacher, and the art of teaching is to structure and exploit such functional influences on the pupils' behaviour. Parents also often set out to change the behaviour of their children by what is essentially a similar procedure, providing occasions when specified patterns of behaviour are reinforced. The exact patterns of behaviour expected of a child at any time are of course determined by the age of the child and by his or her past experience.

Functional analyses of human behaviour are not confined to situations in which discriminative stimuli or reinforcers and punishers are deliberately manipulated by some other person, as by teachers, parents, judges, advisers, therapists or seducers. In less structured situations, as in interactions between friends or strangers for example, the functional context of our behaviour is not normally articulated. Nevertheless, functional analyses may help us to understand better why we do what we do, by alerting us to the ways in which our behaviour may be related to events which have come to acquire functional significance. To take a trite example, our behaviour at parties may differ from our behaviour in supermarkets: parties provide occasions in which accosting another person may be followed by consequences which may be somewhat different from those likely to occur at the check-out desk. More generally, our behaviour may come to be modulated in all sorts of ways by the various environmental circumstances in which we find ourselves.

There is a danger when considering the general approach of functional analyses of behaviour that a picture is painted which is too static or one-sided. A functional account of my behaviour seeks events which set the occasion for and which reinforce or punish my behaviour. Such events, as noted above, are often provided through the behaviour of other people. However, my own behaviour can of course exert similar functional influence over the behaviour of these other people. Thus my behaviour is at one and the same time influenced by and influencing the behaviour of the people with whom I interact through discriminative and reinforcing or punishing effects. It is sometimes difficult to capture this dynamic behavioural interplay when explaining the nature of functional analyses of behaviour, but this *interaction* between the behaviour of people is the very core of this approach to understanding behaviour.

In general, then, functional analyses of behaviour provide a distinctive approach to the study of any pattern of behaviour in any situation. Experimental studies of operant conditioning, often with animal subjects, reveal the ways in which antecedent and consequent events can come to exert a controlling influence on the occurrence of some designated act. Analysis of the functional relationships between these events and behaviour thereby provides an explanatory account of behaviour. Such an account is couched in terms of observable environmental events and manipulable functional relationships between these events and behaviour. The basic principles of the functional analysis of behaviour can be extended to the behaviour of humans. In this case the functionally significant influences on a person's behaviour may be provided by another person, such as a teacher, or indeed by that other person's own behaviour. Functional analyses of human conduct are not limited to structured situations in which one person sets out to influence the behaviour of another. Indeed the approach addresses the dynamic interplay between people which is the very fabric of ordinary social life. In these cases possible functional influences on behaviour must of course be inferred from descriptive accounts of the behavioural repertoires of the individuals in the interaction and the ways in which these repertoires appear to mesh with each other. In all these cases, however, functional analyses of behaviour provide an account of behaviour which is essentially environmentalistic, emphasising how our behaviour can be said to be influenced by what is happening about us rather than by what is happening within us. This is not to deny that people have 'inner lives', whether these be expressed in terms of consciousness or cognitions, or indeed in terms of physiological or neurological processes. The thrust of functional analyses of behaviour, however, is to open up to scrutiny one account of behaviour which, it is claimed, has often been undervalued in psychology, and which may be relevant regardless of the impact of events at other levels. We may now consider how functional analyses may be used in the study of language and verbal behaviour.

Verbal Behaviour

The first point to be made about Skinner's account of language relates
to his very definition of verbal behaviour, said by him to be behaviour
'reinforced through the mediation of other persons' (Skinner, 1957,
p. 2). This definition may appear to be eccentric to the point of being
wilful, for it will be clear that much of the discussion earlier in this
chapter concerning functional analyses of human behaviour is in these
terms about 'verbal behaviour', though it includes no reference to
speech or to the use of words. Skinner's definition has some advantages,
however. In particular, it prepares the way for a *functional* account of
the use of symbols. Symbolic behaviour requires to be interpreted by
another person if it is to have any significance, whereas motor skills,
for example, do not. The distinctive characteristic of 'verbal behaviour'
is therefore said by Skinner to be found in the nature of the *reinforcing
event* which acquires functional control over the behaviour.

One obvious consequence of Skinner's definition is that it includes
gesture and other forms of communication which do not involve the
use of words; indeed, it includes all patterns of social behaviour, not
just those that are described by social psychologists as 'non-verbal communication' (see Chapter 8). Skinner's overt inclusion of physical
gesture in the field of language makes it possible for us to address
immediately the concept of 'meaning', perhaps the most fundamental
issue to be faced by any approach to the study of language. When it is
said that a gesture, or indeed a word, conveys meaning, there seems to
be an implication that meaning exists separately from behaviour. The
question, of course, is *where* that meaning can be thought to exist
before it is conveyed. It seems natural to assume that it might be found
in the mind of the communicator, an assertion that has prompted
MacCorquodale (1969, p. 832) to claim that we have here 'the last
stronghold of mentalism', by which language is made to convey ideas
and meanings which exist in the mind separately and prior to the
expression of the words which are selected to convey them.

A functional account, on the other hand, is reminiscent of the philo-
sophical adage that the meaning of a word is to be found in its usage:
the meaning of a physical gesture is said to be found *within* the functional relationship between that gesture and the behaviour of the
second person who provides reinforcement for it. Thus a wave of the
hand is a physical act which, in certain identifiable circumstances, or
discriminative conditions, leads to certain characteristic consequences
on the part of the audience. A child's wave as a parent is about to leave

prompts characteristic consequences on the part of the parent such as a reciprocal wave (which may itself be reinforced in these circumstances through further waving by the child) or perhaps the utterance 'goodbye'. Waves by the child to other people or in other situations, on the other hand, may be ignored or treated differently. Thus the social world effectively arranges to strengthen the future probability of that act occurring again in similar circumstances, and the gesture can be said to have acquired a communicative function. In turn, the meaning of the verbal utterance 'goodbye', the result of less global physical acts in the use of the vocal system rather than the moving of an arm, can be here analysed in a similar way. Whether with respect to gesture or word, meaning is in general said to be constructed from the functional interaction between the behaviour of two people in certain specified circumstances. Thus 'meaning is not properly regarded as a property either of a response or a situation but rather of the contingencies responsible for both the topography of behavior and the control exerted by stimuli' (Skinner, 1974, p. 90).

Seen in this general light, the task for a theory of verbal behaviour is to emphasise the different possible functional relationships which may influence the occurrence of a gesture or of an utterance. We may develop this idea further by now turning more directly to consider the use of words in speech (i.e., where most theorists might begin their analyses of 'verbal behaviour'). The exposition here will inevitably be only cursory, seeking to convey only the most general principles by means of very simple but fundamental examples.

The first functional class of verbal behaviour discussed by Skinner is termed by him the 'mand', 'a verbal operant in which the response is reinforced by a characteristic consequence and is therefore under the functional control of relevant conditions of deprivation or aversive stimulation' (1957, pp. 35-6). Much of the verbal behaviour of young children is of this sort. Thus the child who cries 'Milk' and is as a result given a drink of milk by a parent can be said to be emitting a mand, for the absence of milk has set the occasion for the response to be followed by this distinctive consequence. Skinner's functional analysis of verbal behaviour does not automatically align itself with traditional grammatical analyses of language, and so an utterance of several words may be deemed functionally equivalent to a single word. Thus, for example, 'Pass the salt' or 'Shut up' may also be mands. The latter utterance provides an example of a mand which occurs in a condition of aversive stimulation (too much noise). A mand may be followed by its characteristic consequence only intermittently, for, as was explained earlier, experimental studies of intermittent reinforcement have demonstrated that behaviour can be sustained at high overall rates by only occasional reinforcement. To move away from the use of words again for a moment, we may notice also that a child's crying may sometimes be functionally identified as a mand (crying when hungry, followed by feeding; crying when wet, followed by change of nappy). Similarly, gestures may be mands, as, for example, with a parent waving a child away when the child is not wanted.

The larger part of verbal behaviour is controlled not by motivational states as are mands but by features of the environment in which we find ourselves. Skinner's second major functional class of verbal behaviour, the 'tact' is defined as 'a verbal operant in which a response of given form is evoked (or at least strengthened) by a particular object or event or property of an object or event' (1957, p. 82). Tacts therefore include utterances which occur in identifiable discriminative conditions and which are then afforded distinctive consequences by others. The naming of objects in the world is a simple example of a tact, one of course which is often deliberately engineered by parents with children: in the presence of an object or a colour, for example, the appropriate verbal behaviour is overtly praised by way of reinforcement. As with our earlier discussion of operant conditioning, however, the reinforcement of a tact may be provided in the natural flow of an unstructured social interaction, as for example when the tact used by one person serves to orientate another to the object concerned. In order to emphasise the functional nature of this analysis, it may be useful to consider once again the single-word utterance 'Milk', discussed above in the context of mands. It should by now be clear to the reader that Skinner's analysis allows for this utterance to have a different function in different environmental conditions: thus the child who cries 'Milk' *when given* a drink of milk is now emitting a tact. This point emphasises that it is not the topography of a response (the muscle movements which cause a particular sound to occur) which forms the unit of analysis here: it is not the word itself which is emphasised in this account, but how it is socially interpreted. Furthermore, the functional significance of an utterance depends on its circumstances and of course on the way in which it is reinforced by others. At the risk of labouring the basic point unduly, we may also note that gestures can be examples of tacts, as for example when a child points to 'all the green animals'. Crying, too, can be a tact as well as a mand. Tacts form a significant part of verbal behaviour, for their controlling relations are 'nothing less than the whole of the physical environment – the world of things and events which a speaker is said to "talk about" ' (Skinner, 1957, p. 81).

Skinner's account of verbal behaviour includes other functional classes which are under different forms of discriminative control, including 'echoic' speech which 'generates a sound pattern similar to the stimulus' (1957, p. 55) and 'textual operants' which are vocal responses 'under the control of a nonauditory verbal stimulus' (1957, p. 66), such as written or printed material (including pictures). These and other classes of verbal behaviour are all defined solely in functional terms, their provenance and 'meaning' emerging from their setting conditions and their consequences, i.e. from their environmental and social context. Skinner's account also includes classes of words, such as 'auto-clitics' (1957, p. 311), which may be said to serve a more convention-ally grammatical function, allowing the development of sequences of functional units. It is not possible here to develop these aspects of his systematic approach (see Skinner, 1957). However, the basic concept of a functional analysis of language may by now have emerged satis-factorily, thus allowing us to consider some of its implications.

Some Ramifications of the Functional Analysis of Language

Skinner's approach to the study of 'verbal behaviour' is a sustained extension of his theoretical approach to psychology as a whole. The burden of his system is to explain behaviour in terms of its functional relationships with environmental events which may serve as discrimina-tive stimuli by setting the occasion for emission of specific acts, or which may serve as reinforcers or punishers and modulate the fre-quency of those acts. The system is both environmentalistic and deter-ministic, that is to say it emphasises that the causes of behaviour are to be found in its environmental context. The extension of this approach to 'verbal behavour' is accomplished by focusing on human behaviour whose frequency is modulated by reinforcement or punishment provided by other members of what Skinner terms the verbal com-munity.

Even in its most general context, Skinner's system has seemed controversial and even austere to many commentators, principally because of its emphasis on environmental influences on behaviour. This radical behaviourist perspective places little emphasis on the traditional autonomy of individuals to act as they choose, and the attribution of the responsibility for our actions to our social environment has profound general implications which Skinner has considered in his book *Beyond Freedom and Dignity* (1972a).

In the domain of language, the approach is certainly challenging to our normal preconceptions. We saw that a rat is said to press a lever in an operant conditioning experiment *because* a light acts as a discriminative stimulus and *because* of the selective effects of reinforcement on that act. By extension, the artist utters the tact 'That's a Picasso' *because* a specific painting provides a discriminative stimulus and *because* the act has in the past been reinforced by social mediation when it has occurred in appropriate circumstances. The traditional ascription of autonomy of human action is thereby challenged even in the area of language, which seems most persistently to demand that a distinction be drawn between behaviour and the person who is behaving, thereby allowing for speech to reflect autonomous inner processes and allowing us to say 'what we want to say'. Skinner has not shrunk from the impact of this point. In a provocative paper entitled 'On having a poem' (1972b) he has gone so far as to assert that emphasising the creativity of a poet deflects us from understanding the poet's role as a locus or place where environmental influences come together in a way which is potentially open to public scrutiny to produce the novel strings of words which we call a poem. The 'having' of a poem by a poet in this sense is likened to the having of a baby by a woman; in both cases the 'agent' is in effect simply a place where processes which can be understood scientifically come together, and although the product is novel and unique, the ascription of praise or blame for the creativity is tempered.

Such an analysis of the richest aspects of human behaviour is bound to provoke controversy and perhaps some misunderstanding. MacCorquodale (1970) has suggested that it was the impact of conclusions such as the above which may have been partly responsible for the famous critique of Skinner's account of verbal behaviour produced by Chomsky (1959). Chomsky offered three main criticisms, which are reviewed by MacCorquodale. First, it is argued that Skinner's functional analyses of verbal behaviour are no more than untested hypotheses. Second, the approach is said to gain spurious scientific rigour from the illegitimate and even casual generalisation of scientific concepts appropriate to the conditioning laboratory to inappropriate settings such as those in which we live and interact with others. Chomsky's critique is somewhat blunted here by the fact that he seems not to have recognised the full force of the functional approach which is being extrapolated. For example, he repeatedly implies that reinforcement is thought by Skinner to reduce some drive or need, an interpretation of reinforcement which is out of place in Skinner's system and which is used in the very different theoretical context of Hullian learning theory, with which Skinner's theoretical account of behaviour has been in constant competition (see Hilgard and Bower, 1975). Similarly Chomsky fails to appreciate that stimuli and responses are defined in Skinner's system solely in terms of their functional relationships with each other — an event cannot be defined as a discriminative stimulus without its being functionally related to behaviour, and in turn behaviour cannot be defined as a response unless its functional relationship with a consequence has been identified. Thus, in both the simple operant conditioning experiment and the analysis of verbal behaviour, discriminative stimuli, operant responses and reinforcers are defined solely in terms of identifiable functional relationships between them in given situations, and not in terms of any intrinsic qualities which they may have.

The third major point made by Chomsky is that speech is complex and can therefore only be understood by means of complex mediational or neurological accounts. It is this view which has led to the emphasis in psycholinguistics on grammatical structures which make possible the emergence of novel but meaningful sentences. With respect to the provenance of verbal behaviour (as opposed to its structural characteristics), Chomsky expressed the opinion that 'in the present state of our knowledge, we must attribute an overwhelming influence on actual behavior to ill-defined factors of attention, set, volition and caprice' (1959, p. 30). Such a view is in striking contrast to the programme which Skinner set himself of seeking an account of human language which was similar in principle to the deterministic analyses of other patterns of behaviour which were beginning to emerge from experimental studies of operant conditioning.

It must of course be admitted that functional analyses can not in fact deal at an empirical level with the richness and unpredictability of most human language — although the extent to which some aspects of our everyday verbal repertoires are predictable and understandable in these terms can be underplayed. An important additional concept here in Skinner's account of verbal behaviour is that of multiple causation. The momentary strength of a single verbal utterance is usually a function of more than one variable, as we have already seen in the discussion above about how 'Milk' can be functionally determined as a mand or as a tact (or indeed, of course, as an echoic or a textual response). Thus very different environmental contexts can lead to the occurrence of the same topographical pattern of behaviour. On the other hand, a single environmental variable can often affect the future probability of more than one response. For example, Skinner (1957, p. 227) notes that 'the adult repertoire contains many mands varying with one state of deprivation . . . ; when a man is deprived of food, it is not simply the mand "Food!" which shows an increased probability'. A complete functional analysis of verbal behaviour could only be successful if the whole past history of these functional relationships can be unravelled for each individual – an unrealistic empirical programme. The most important point here, however, is that Skinner is striving to develop a system in which even human verbal behaviour can *in principle* be understood in terms of functional relationships between behaviour and environmental events.

It should not be thought that functional analysis has no place whatever for 'private events' occurring within us. In fact Skinner has developed some particularly interesting discussions about the ways in which we come to talk about, and indeed experience, events within our skin which are by their very nature not amenable to scrutiny by other members of our verbal community (see, for example, Skinner, 1957, pp. 130-8; 1974, pp. 137-88). We may consider here the ways in which we may come to tact such private stimuli. As Skinner notes, if we are able to talk about such things as heartburn or boredom, a functional analysis of such tacts requires the designation of an appropriate discriminative stimulus. However, our verbal community cannot itself have access to our private experiences in order to reinforce an utterance appropriately in the way that it does with tacts prompted by objects or events in the external world. In such cases, Skinner suggests, the verbal community has to make its best efforts to deal with these verbal operants by reference to the broader behavioural context. If a child complains of a pain, for example, parents can have no way of sharing the experience directly, and so they must therefore seek collateral evidence to allow them to make a decision about how to reinforce the apparent tact – is the 'painful' area inflamed or damaged?; is the context appropriately supportive (i.e., could the child be thought to be malingering for 'other reasons')?; does the child's overt behaviour show supportive signs, such as squirming? In this way the verbal community may do its best to teach the experience of pain in a way similar to that used to teach the experience of green. The fact that this can of necessity be done only indirectly, however, provides a reason for the fact that our language about inner experiences and emotions is often so much less precise and more diffuse than is our language concerning the world about us.

We are now beginning to delve into quite difficult, perhaps even esoteric, issues in the functional analysis of verbal behaviour. The intention here is simply to indicate that the system is more coherent and extensive than critics sometimes imply. The attempt to handle language at a theoretical level by means of systematic principles derived from the psychological laboratory should not perhaps be too readily dismissed as crude and insensitive, and the crucial importance of identifying potentially significant *relationships* between behaviour and environmental events should not be overlooked, as has so often been done by critics of Skinner's approach such as Chomsky. This point is important because the extension of the theory to admittedly difficult empirical and conceptual issues in the domain of language can be said to provide a context for more specific language remediation programmes which are based on similar principles. It is surely important to consider carefully how far language can be understood in ways similar to those which have proved useful with respect to other behavioural problems.

Conclusion

The aim of this chapter is to suggest that what a person *says* may in principle be amenable to a behavioural analysis which is essentially similar to that which has proved effective in helping us to understand in other contexts why people *do* what they do. Verbal behaviour is effected, like all patterns of behaviour, by means of the controlled use of muscles, in this case the vocal musculature mentioned in the quotation with which this chapter opened. Behavioural interventions in language remediation programmes use techniques of operant conditioning in order to teach people how to use these muscles more effectively, and other chapters in this book review some of these approaches more extensively. Behavioural programmes can also be used to attempt to help people 'use language' more effectively and appropriately, and this approach is also reviewed in subsequent chapters. The present chapter attempts to supplement these contributions by providing a broader context for these forms of remediative work. Behavioural analyses have a role to play in helping us to understand language in general. The functional analyses of contemporary behaviourism thereby have the unusual virtue of providing a framework for the study of all aspects of language and language remediation.

References

Blackman, D.E. (1974) *Operant Conditioning: an Experimental Analysis of Behaviour*, Methuen, London

Chomsky, N. (1959) 'Verbal Behavior', by B.F. Skinner, *Language, 35*, 26-58

Davey, G. (1981) *Animal Learning and Conditioning*, Macmillan, London.

Hilgard, E.R. and Bower, G.H. (1975) *Theories of Learning* (4th ed.), Prentice-Hall, Englewood Cliffs, New Jersey

MacCorquodale, K. (1969) B.F. Skinner's *Verbal Behavior:* a retrospective appreciation, *Journal of the Experimental Analysis of Behavior, 12*, 831-41

——(1970) On Chomsky's review of Skinner's *Verbal Behavior, Journal of the Experimental Analysis of Behavior, 13*, 83-99

Skinner, B.F. (1957) *Verbal Behavior*, Appleton-Century-Crofts, New York

——(1972a) *Beyond Freedom and Dignity*, Knopf, New York

——(1972b) A lecture on 'having a poem', in B.F. Skinner, *Cumulative Record* (3rd ed.), Appleton-Century-Crofts, New York

——(1974) *About Behaviorism*, Knopf, New York

2 BEHAVIOURAL APPROACHES TO TREATING LANGUAGE DISORDERS

Donald E. Mowrer

In the initial section of this chapter, I will attempt to sketch out the basic principles of behaviourism as applied to the acquisition and maintenance of human behaviour. Next I will review the literature illustrating how these principles have been utilised to modify language behaviours. Finally, I will evaluate the present status of the behavioural approach to learning. This is not meant to negate the importance of other theories such as mediational and cognitive approaches that offer alternative explanations of language acquisition.

Basic Principles of The Behavioural Approach

Behaviourism is bound by a simple principle — that human behaviour is lawful. Proponents of behaviourism seek to discover functional relationships between independent variables and response classes through systematic analysis. Once these relationships are determined, it is possible to make effective predictions and modifications of behaviour. Attention is focused upon events that can be observed and measured precisely. Kanfer and Phillips (1970) review five components important to the behavioural model: stimuli, organism, response, response-consequence contingency, and consequence.

Stimuli

Environmental conditions that have a functional relationship to behaviour comprise the stimulus component. Discriminative stimuli (S^D) are those that signal a high probability that a response will be reinforced while stimuli signalling no reinforcement which follow a response are called non-discriminative stimuli (S^Δ). Discriminative stimuli can be produced by other persons or they may consist of self-induced stimuli.

Organism

The biological state of the organism is important since different biological states can greatly alter behavioural responses. Presence of toxic substances, disease, drugs, chromosomal deficiencies, nutritional deficiencies, and so on, are some of the variables that can influence behaviour.

Response

Lindsley (1964) describes behaviour in terms of a movement that has a definite beginning and ending. Most learning theorists differentiate between two response classes:

(a) involuntary (respondent) responses associated with classical conditioning are modified as a result of continguous association of two stimuli; and

(b) voluntary (operant) responses associated with instrumental conditioning are modified by the consequences following the responses. Some psychologists question the value of making this dichotomy between voluntary and involuntary behaviour but for classification purposes, the distinction is a useful one (Rescorla and Solomon, 1967).

Response-consequence Contingency

This variable deals with the arrangement between behaviour and its consequences; that is, how frequently reinforcement follows responses. Data from human and animal research demonstrate differential effects of various schedules of reinforcement upon speed of acquisition, strength of response and delay of established responses.

Consequence

The consequence of a response is an important ingredient of the operant conditioning model. If the immediate consequence of a response serves to increase the probability a response will occur in the future, the consequence is defined as a reinforcing stimulus. The effectiveness of a consequence varies considerably from person to person. If the consequence serves to decrease response frequency, it is called a punisher.

These five elements are the basic components of study in the behavioural approach to learning. Behaviour is explained by the unique functional relationship among these elements. All elements can be defined objectively, measured and manipulated. The goal of behaviourism is to predict and control behaviour in much the same way as physicists and biologists predict and control events in the natural sciences.

Behavioural Conditioning

Learning can be defined as a change in behaviour brought about by experience. Early in the 1920s, Pavlov used the term conditioning to designate a specific type of learning. He studied the effects of manipulating the first three behavioural elements: the stimulus event, the biological state of the organism and the response. His demonstration of *classical or respondent conditioning* was accomplished by the frequent pairing of an unconditioned stimulus or UCS (meat powder) with a conditioned stimulus CS (tone). As a result of the frequent stimulus pairing, the organism's response (CR) to the conditional stimulus (CS) becomes very similar to the original response to the unconditional stimulus. Administering consequences plays no role in respondent conditioning. Also, classical conditioning cannot be used to establish a new response. It only pairs a new stimulus to an old one. It is usually assumed that respondent conditioning involves changes in the glands, smooth muscles, or other physiological systems outside voluntary control. The clinical application of respondent conditioning is usually found in aversion therapies aimed at eliminating sexual-deviances, alcoholism and enuresis. It has also been used to demonstrate how neurotic symptoms such as fetishes and phobias are acquired. The acquisition of attitudes, feelings and emotional responses may be the result of classical conditioning. If stimuli are associated with pleasant events (smiling, happy people), our attitude toward the stimulus is favourable. But if we associate stimuli with unpleasant events (shock) we avoid the conditional stimulus. An association is made between two stimuli, the conditional stimulus and the unconditional stimulus, when one stimulus is contingent upon the other.

Starkweather (1983) points out classical conditioning often occurs simultaneously with instrumental conditioning. For example, when a teacher frequently rewards a child for a correct response, the teacher (CS) and the reward (US) become associated and the child is conditioned to respond to the teacher (CS) in a positive manner (CR). When this occurs, the teacher can fade out tangible rewards and substitute smiles and attention. In this manner, it is possible to establish new stimulus control over certain response classes.

Another example parallels Pavlov's experiment. Assuming an infant salivates when milk is presented, the parent says 'milk', then presents milk to the infant, after which the infant salivates. After several 'milk'-milk pairings, the infant salivates when the parent says 'milk'. The infant reacts to the spoken word milk in a similar manner as to the real milk. The infant has been conditioned to respond to a word as a symbol for a specific referant.

A second type of conditioning, called *instrumental or operant conditioning*, focuses upon the last three behavioural components, namely the response, the response-consequence contingency and the consequence. In contrast to classical conditioning in which association between stimuli is emphasised, the consequence of the response is the focal point in instrumental conditioning. Instrumental conditioning is considered as the only appropriate method for modifying voluntary and skeletal-muscle behaviours (Kanfer and Phillips, 1970). However, there is evidence to demonstrate achievement of operant control over autonomic processes as well (Grings and Carlin, 1966; Helmer and Furedy, 1968).

Efforts clearly to separate classical from instrumental conditioning models have not been entirely successful. While emphasis may be placed upon stimulus or consequence elements in a learning situation, we must be aware of the fact that complex human functioning involves parameters of all aspects of the behavioural model. Often both classical and instrumental conditioning may be operating concurrently.

The critical difference between the two types of conditioning is that during classical conditioning, reinforcement is present every time the stimulus is presented but during instrumental conditioning, reinforcement is presented only following specified responses. The experimenter determines which response will be followed by a reward during instrumental conditioning. In considering a theoretical example of how a child might be instrumentally conditioned to say a word, first we assume a motivational state exists within the child. Suppose the child is thirsty. Assume also, as shown in Figure 2.1, that the child can produce several verbal utterances (R_n). Each time 'wa-wa' (R_4) is uttered, water (S^R) is presented. Water is not presented following other responses (R_1, R_2, R_3). After several trials, the child becomes conditioned to say 'wa-wa' when thirsty, not 'pe-pe', 'lo-lo' or 'bye-bye'. The desire for water is the stimulus that evokes the response 'wa-wa', the presentation of water is the *positive reinforcer*. The important feature involved in establishing a verbal operant rests with the consequence of the behaviour (Skinner, 1957). If, in the previous example, the listener produces water, the positive reinforcer, following the utterance 'lo-lo' (as would be the case if the parent was French-speaking) but not

Figure 2.1: Model of Operant Conditioning of Response 'wa-wa' in Presence of Thirsty Condition

Motivational State	Possible Response	Listener Response
Thirsty (Possibly sight of water)	R_1 'pe-pe' R_2 'lo-lo' R_3 'bye-bye' R_4 'wa-wa' $\vdots$ R_n	LR_a Presentation of water LR_b Silence

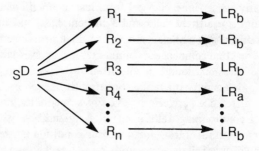

following 'wa-wa (S^Δ), then 'lo-lo' (S^D) would be the conditional response since its utterance results in water, the desired consequence.

This example demonstrating how a child might be conditioned to say 'wa-wa' when thirsty is used to illustrate the process of operant conditioning. Obviously, if parents waited for appropriate verbal responses or even approximations to occur before administering reinforcement, it is doubtful children would ever learn language. By providing verbal prompts, we can shorten the child's trial-and-error search for the correct utterances. Prompts were used extensively to evoke responses in the early research demonstrating operant conditioning of verbal responses (Sloane and MacAulay, 1968). A common procedure consists of three temporal events: present a picture or an object to the child, such as a ball; state 'Say ball'; and provide a reinforcer contingent upon the child's appropriate imitative response. With continual practice, the child is conditioned to name objects when requested. No reinforcement is provided for incorrect responses. The important feature of operant conditioning is that the response is instrumental in acquiring the desired event.

Negative reinforcement (see D in Table 2.1), a second procedure for increasing response rate, is almost never used to change language behaviours. Its use is limited to individuals whose behaviour is considered extremely deviant. First, an aversive stimulus such as shock or a loud noise is presented. When the organism makes the desired response, the aversive stimulus is terminated. If the desired response increases in frequency it is said to be negatively reinforced. For example, the wife who nags her husband to perform chores in the home illustrates how negative reinforcement can be used to control the husband's behaviour. In order to terminate the nagging behaviour (the negative reinforcer) he performs the chores.

Altering consequences of behaviour plays a key role in determining whether response rate increases or decreases. If an unpleasant or aversive stimulus is presented following a particular response, the likelihood this response will occur in the future under similar conditions is decreased. This condition, called *punishment*, is shown in Table 2.1B. Lovaas (1968) used punishment in the form of a loud, stern 'no', or slap on the hand to suppress inattentive, self-destructive, and tantrum behaviours.

Unfortunately, punishment usually has only a temporary effect upon behaviour rates and may result in undesirable side-effects that may retard establishment of desired behaviours. Sometimes the mere attention one receives during punishment may itself be more reinforcing than the punishment procedure itself and this is ineffective in decelerating behaviours. Punishment in mild forms, such as the use of verbal statements like 'no' and 'wrong', has been found to be very useful in helping the individual identify the undesirable behaviour. These mild forms are swift, contingent upon specific behaviours, and can be administered according to a variety of schedules.

Response cost is another punishment procedure whereby reinforcers are withdrawn contingent upon undesirable behaviours. This procedure is effective especially when all members of a peer group lost privileges as a result of one child's misbehaviour. However, McReynolds and Huston (1970) concluded response cost was not an effective procedure in articulation therapy when token loss equalled or surpassed token gain.

A fourth procedure, *extinction* (Table 2.1C), involves removal of

Table 2.1: Four Types of Instrument Conditioning Specified by Consequences of Behaviour

	Presentation of Stimulus	Removal of Stimulus
Rewarding Stimulus	**A** Positive Reinforcement	**C** Extinction
Aversive Stimulus	**B** Punishment	**D** Negative Reinforcement (Escape)

reinforcers to produce decrements in behaviour. If the reward used to condition a response is removed, the frequency of the conditional response increases briefly, then gradually decreases to its preconditioned rate. In some instances, the child's behaviour may be so disruptive that it is best to remove the child to a separate room or area where there is no opportunity to receive reinforcement for the behaviour. The term *time-out* (TO) is used to describe this type of isolation and has been used frequently with children who exhibit tantrums, excessive crying, or destructive behaviours that detract from their learning or the learning of others. Time-out can take the form of simply looking away from the child when mild disruptive behaviour occurs. Risley and Wolf (1968) used this time-out procedure to decrease chanting and shrieking behaviours in an autistic child. Inadvertently, chanting and shrieking behaviours were conditioned to a high rate. Parents were advised to turn away from the child when chanting occurred. When chanting changed to shrieking, the child was taken to a room for a five-minute period. Every attempt was made to remove attention (reinforcement) following chanting or screaming. After the removal of reinforcers, chanting and shrieking behaviours decreased to their preconditioned rate, that is, they were extinguished.

Behaviourists stress the importance consequences play in determining behaviour rates. Baer and Wolf (1968) state that *what* the teacher does is not nearly so important as *when* it is done. This simple principle, making teacher behaviours contingent upon specific child behaviours, is the essence of behaviour modifications. Results of numerous studies that focus upon manipulation of consequence events confirm the notion that one who controls consequences of a behaviour can control the rate of that behaviour. As Bijou (1970, p. 68) states, 'Teaching . . . is a situation in which the teacher arranges the contingencies of reinforcement to expedite learning by the child'.

In summary two techniques are used in operant conditioning models to increase behaviour rates (positive and negative reinforcement) and two are used to decrease behaviour rates (punishment and extinction). Several variations of these procedures will be discussed in this chapter.

Evoking Behaviours

Antecedent events have been manipulated in many ways to evoke the desired response. In many cases the objective was to alter an existing speech response but occasionally, as is the case with the nonverbal child, there is no speech response to modify. Establishing new responses has been accomplished successfully through a process of *shaping* the response. Antecedent events often play an important role in shaping new responses. The most common technique is to provide a verbal prompt by telling the individual what to say or do.

Arranging the environment to increase the likelihood the desired response will occur constitutes a second technique. Removing all stimuli except the desired stimulus often forces the child to attend to the stimulus. A third procedure is manually to assist the individual in making the response. This can be done by shaping the lips to assist one in producing the desired sound. This procedure was utilised by Lovaas (1968), in teaching a psychotic child how to produce [b]. The experimenter held the child's lips together using fingers and quickly removed them when the child exhaled. A fourth and commonly used prompt is to provide a model for the child to imitate. McKenna-Hartung and Hartung (1973) illustrated the use of this technique to establish verbal imitation skills in autistic children. Children were rewarded only if they emited a sound within the prescribed time after the adult presented the model.

Consequent events also are important in shaping behaviour. Once a response has been evoked, the next step is to increase the frequency of that response. This is done by providing reinforcement immediately following the desired response. Often a child's response does not match the target response exactly. In this case it is essential to evoke a number of responses so only those closely approximating the desired response are reinforced. Others are extinguished by withholding reinforcement. This process of shaping through *differential reinforcement* (reinforcing successive approximations) makes it possible to teach new responses not available previously. Sherman (1965) described this process in teaching a 63-year-old mute patient to imitate the word 'food'. At first, the patient produced indistinguishable mumbles and grunts. Only responses similar to a prolonged [u] were reinforced. The responses similar to [u d] were reinforced and finally responses close to 'food' were reinforced. After 25 sessions the subject was correctly repeating 12 additional words as a result of this shaping process.

As the behaviour is strengthened, prompts are gradually removed or *faded* until they are no longer necessary (Risley and Wolf, 1968). Finally, the goal is to bring the behaviour under control of natural reinforcement contingencies in the person's environment. Often difficulties are encountered in shaping behaviour because the steps are not made small enough for the individual to achieve success or adequate prompts are not utilised.

Selecting Reinforcers

Usually, food items have been used as an effective reinforcer in many operant conditioning studies that attempt to teach speech. Actually, a large number of other reinforcers can be used. Birnbrauer, Burchard, and Burchard (1970) suggest five ways one might select potential reinforcers. The simplest procedure is simply ask the individual for a list of preferences or allow the person to choose from a group of pre-selected items that have been found to be reinforcing to others. The items may consist of various toys attached to a posterboard or a list of activities (Addison and Homme, 1966).

A second method of selecting a reinforcer involves observing the individual's behaviour. Those behaviours that occur most frequently where choice is allowed will usually serve as reinforcers for behaviours that occur infrequently. If, for example, a child sketches when given the opportunity but avoids reading, then opportunity to sketch may be used as a reinforcer for reading (Ayllon and Azrin, 1968). This technique is similar to reinforcement sampling in which the individual is observed selecting reinforcers in a free play situation.

One should never underestimate the power of adult or peer attention as a reinforcer. This third potential reinforcer frequently is used in the classroom settings and consists of positive verbal statements, body contact, visual contact, close proximity and applauding. Fourth, one can select items that are highly valued by peers, such as high sugar content food items, crayons, toys, games, excursions and privileges. Many severely retarded, psychotic, or autistic children do not share these preferences hence it is difficult to find effective reinforcers for them.

For most individuals tokens can be used as effective reinforcers. Points, poker chips, stars or check marks are provided contingent upon the described behaviour. These tokens can be exchanged for a variety of other reinforcers. They have the following advantages: they are easily administered, not consumable, and can be exchanged for other items (Girardeau and Spradlin, 1970a).

Techniques for Maintaining Behaviours

B.F. Skinner discovered almost by accident early in the 1930s that when rats were given only one pellet per minute, no matter how many times they pressed the lever, their rate of responding was considerably higher than when every press was reinforced (Rachlin, 1970). This finding ran contrary to the notion that the greater the amount of reinforcement the greater the amount of responding. Generally, continuous reinforcement is required to establish a new behaviour but once learned the behaviour can be maintained at high rates by intermittent reinforcement.

The effects of using different reinforcement schedules have been studied extensively in the laboratory both with humans and animals. Fixed ratio schedules produce an extremely high rate of responding with only a slight post-reinforcement pause. Such a schedule is found in jobs where the employee must produce a fixed number of products to receive a reinforcer. The child who receives a reward each time three words are uttered is on a fixed-ratio 3 (responses) to 1 (reward). Reinforcement can be delivered following certain time periods (fixed-interval). If a reward is given every two minutes, the schedule is said to be a fixed-interval 2 minutes. Fixed ratio and interval schedules are not common in the natural environment but have been used in many language training programmes.

Examples of variable ratio and interval schedules, on the other hand, abound in everyday situations. The pay-off of a slot machine is a good example of the variable-ratio schedule. The more coins you insert, the greater the likelihood of a pay-off but one never knows how many coins will be required to receive the pay-off. As with fixed-ratio schedules, extremely high response rates will occur under variable-ratio schedules. Variable-interval schedules also result in a high constant rate of response, but not to the degree variable-ratio schedules generate. Behaviours reinforced on variable-ratio schedules are often extremely resistant to extinction. This explains why some behaviours persist in spite of the fact no reinforcement seems forthcoming.

Response Chaining

A response chain is a series of isolated responses that have been conditioned to occur in sequence. Many behaviourists contend sentences are simply strings of words in which the first word triggers the second word, that word triggers a third and so on. Animal experiments clearly demonstrated how these chains could be conditioned by teaching a sequence of complex motor behaviours, such as climbing a spiral stair, crossing a bridge, climbing a ladder, and so on, finally attaining a food pellet (Pierrel and Sherman, 1963). Sidman (1965), demonstrated how severely retarded children were conditioned upon sight of the therapist to stop other activities, go to a certain location, sit in a circle with other children, wait until a ball is rolled to them, roll the ball back, and receive a token that they could exchange for a toy three to six hours later (cited in Kanfer and Phillips, 1970). Children have been taught many self-help behaviours, such as dressing themselves, toileting and bathing

Gray and Ryan (1971) used backward chaining in teaching proper grammatical sequences to children. The child is shown a blue ball. The clinician models the sentence 'Johnny, the ball is blue. Johnny, is blue.' The child is expected to repeat 'is blue'. Next 'ball is blue' is modelled and repeated and finally 'the ball is blue' is the target response.

Observing and Measuring Behaviours

Change that occurs in the frequency of behaviour reflects the efficacy of behaviour modification procedures. Behaviourists give particular attention to precise descriptions and measurements of the target behaviour and its rate changes. Mentalistic concepts that cannot be discretely measured have no place in the behavioural approach. Direct observation of environmental stimuli and rate changes are essential ingredients of behavioural modification programmes.

First, the behaviour to be modified must be observable and measurable. Much of the literature in education deals with observation of behaviours important to learning. Such behaviours include attention, seat-leaving, co-operation, speaking, reading, problem solving description, and the like. Behaviours are counted in discrete units so one can determine whether they increase or decrease during the observational period. The behaviour must have an observable beginning and ending. Behaviourists who study verbal behaviours employ numerous means of analysing language samples. The simplest procedure is to count the number of times a specific response occurs. Lovaas (1968), for example, counted single sounds emitted by psychotic children during the first step of his training programme. Next he recorded syllables, then words categorising them as nouns, prepositions, pronouns and other parts of speech. Length of utterance is an observable measure used by Risley, Reynolds and Hart (1970), who counted words spoken in response to questions asked by the teacher. They also counted the number of different words used, frequency of child-initiated conversation, complexity of narratives, appropriate use of adjectives, spontaneous speech attempts, verbal statements pertaining to the child's activities and attitudes, and verbal interchanges between children and parents. Verbal behaviours are classified, counted and related to antecedent and/or consequent events that occur in the child's environment.

Johnston and Harris (1968) present detailed instructions concerning how to select, classify, observe and record verbal behaviours. They stress the importance of making reliable and valid observations using two or more observers. Unless accurate and systematic observations are made, little is learned from experimentation. Birnbrauer, Burchard and Burchard (1970) illustrated the importance of keeping accurate data in their description of a classroom teacher who made subjective judgements about rate changes in students. Like most of us, the teacher was unresponsive to small increments in behaviour but alert only to large changes in behaviour rates. Using teaching method A she observed no astounding rate changes according to her subjective measurement. Consequently, she tried methods, B, C D and E during the ensuing weeks all producing what she considered as meagre results. Finally she concluded that her class was hopeless as none of the methods worked well. But had she carefully observed behaviour rates daily several days in succession, she might have observed a trend to show one of the methods produced the desired behavioural change.

Skinner (1966) was meticulous in his measurement of animal behaviour rates. Responses were defined in terms of overt actions such as lever or button presses. Each response is recorded by a cumulative recorder 24 hours a day for months on end! But even the best laid plans can go wrong. Skinner (1966) describes how he discovered extinction curves because of a jammed mechanism that failed to disperse food pellets to a pigeon during the night. Observation of the recorded pecking responses the following morning produced a response extinction curve uncorrupted by the physiological process of ingestion.

Another important aspect of observation in behavioural experiments involves methodological design. To demonstrate the effect of certain variations upon behaviour, an ABA reversal design usually is employed. First the behaviour is observed over time (condition A) until it appears the behaviour rate is stable (baseline). An experimental variable is introduced (condition B) and its effect upon the target behaviour is observed. Then the experimental variable is withdrawn to re-establish the original condition (condition A). If the rate of behaviour changes under condition B but returns to the baseline level during condition A, then it can be argued that the introduction of the experimental variable was solely responsible for the change of behaviour. There are several variations of this design. Some prefer an ABAB design in which the experimental variable (condition B) is reinstated. A second variable can be added to produce an ABACA design.

Sometimes it is not appropriate to use these designs when studying acquisition of verbal behaviours. Often, newly learned language responses are maintained by the child's environment because, from a functional standpoint, use of the newly learned behaviour can result in reinforcement outside the experimental condition. When it is not possible to reverse a condition, a *multiple baseline* technique can be used (Risley and Baer, 1973).

This technique utilises two or more behaviours that are measured concurrently. After baseline is taken, the experimental variable is introduced first to only one of the behaviours. Behaviour rates are compared with changes that may occur in a second or third behaviour under observation. If no changes are noted in the other behaviours but change is noted in the first behaviour, it is concluded this change is a result of the introduction of the experimental variable. In spite of these rigorous attempts to control the effects of error, Hanley (1970) points out these techniques do not automatically guarantee the variables under study are directly responsible for behavioural change.

Application of the Behavioural Approach in the Treatment of Language Disorders

The behavioural approach is a process used to change a behaviour based upon observable events as opposed to mentalistic concepts. The key techniques used to modify behaviour lie in the antecedent and consequent events that precede and follow the response. Reinforcement is the heart of the operant conditioning paradigm and is used to strengthen behaviour, gradually to shape new responses, to build long and complex response chains, and to bring behaviour under stimulus control. Language is viewed as an operant behaviour that can be taught by manipulating stimulus events to evoke imitative responses that can be shaped and maintained using appropriate schedules of reinforcement.

One of the earliest attempts to explain a learning theory of language was set forth in Miller and Dollard's (1941) text. Language acquisition was considered to follow the same principles of learning as other forms of social behaviour. Children learn speech by imitating their parents who in turn provide rewards for speech attempts. Words are mastered and strung together in proper sequence by trial and error. Parents serve as models and provide correction of grammatical errors until the child eventually masters language.

This simplistic approach was expanded upon by Skinner (1957) in his book *Verbal Behavior*. Skinner's learning theory approach to language provided the foundation for most behavioural approaches to the treatment of language problems during the following two decades. For Skinner, stimulus, response and reinforcement were the important elements in the study of language learning. Verbal responses are conditioned to occur by providing reinforcement under specified stimulus conditions. If a ball is presented and the child responds 'ball', reinforcement often follows, that is, parents nod or give the ball to the child. Frequently such occurrences strengthen the ball-naming response when a ball is presented. Skinner identified six major verbal operants (mand, echoic, textual, intraverbal, tact and autoclitic) and explained how each was used in a language context. He also discussed thinking as a type of covert verbal behaviour where the speaker provides self reinforcement. Skinner's work had an important impact upon the views of those who were responsible for treating language disorders.

As a result of Skinner's theory some speech/language pathologists began to take an interest in using a behavioural approach as a technique for teaching language to retarded and autistic children. At the time, there was little information concerning how to deal with children whose language was nonexistent or severely delayed. Barely 20 articles appeared in the *Journal of Speech and Language Disorders* between 1936-61 concerning the topic of language disorders. Five times the number of articles appeared under the heading of articulation disorders, while ten times as many articles were written about stuttering.

One of the first articles calling the attention of speech/language pathologists to merits of the behavioural approach appeared in 1961 (Shelton, Arndt and Miller, 1961). The authors sketched out basic components of the operant conditioning model emphasising the importance of reinforcement as a potentially powerful tool clinicians could use to modify communication behavours. They discussed the importance of contiguity between response and reward, the use of intermittent reinforcement, and the repression of responses through extinction. Curiously, they also discussed the importance of insight, a concept rejected by most avid behaviourists. Nevertheless, the concepts suggested in this article represented a departure from the traditional approaches used in the treatment of language disorders. During the next decade, several articles were written that clearly identified the basic principles of operant conditioning as applied to speech pathology (Brookshire, 1967; Holland, 1967; Girardeau and Spradlin, 1970b; and McReynolds, 1970).

One of the first reports concerning use of a behavioural approach in treating language disorders was published in the 1963 *Journal of Speech and Hearing Disorders* monograph. The rationale for the research studies reported in this monograph were based upon the following assumptions (Schiefelbusch, 1963, p. 5)

The study of language and communcation will be facilitated if the terms are defined so that events to which they refer can be observed, classified, and measured, that is, defined operationally.

Language and communication behavior is determined by other events which can be objectively described, classified, and in many instances, manipulated.

Language behavior is learned and as such is subject to the same principles as other behaviors.

The research setting for studies reported in this monograph, was a residential institution for retarded individuals in Parsons, Kansas. The major topics included in this monograph were: the development of a language test, an analysis of interpersonal language behaviours between two levels of mentally retarded children and adults, and the effects of type and percentage of reinforcement on the acquisition and extinction of a complex verbal task. The studies demonstrated the feasibility of using an operant conditioning paradigm to identify important learner variables related to language acquisition. Language behaviour was defined as observable verbal responses. It was shown that verbal responses could be increased or decreased by systematically manipulating consequences. Another group of studies focused upon amount of verbal output as a function of adult expectations, a pragmatic language function. It wasn't until the late 1970s that researchers seriously began to study these pragmatic aspects of language.

It is important to understand the trend of research in language prior to the 1963 JSHD monograph if one is to follow the course of the behaviouristic movement in the treatment of language disorders. The early classic studies of McCarthy (1930), Day (1932) and Davis (1937) highlighted the detrimental effects lower social class, institutionalisation of infants and minority membership have on language development. Numerous subsequent studies verified these early findings, namely that absence of or inadequate verbally-oriented interactions between adults and children can have lasting and harmful effects upon language development (Fleming, 1942; Goldfarb, 1945; Brown, 1944; Brodbeck and Irwin, 1946; Pasamanick, 1946; Hunt, 1961; Fowler, 1962).

Impoverished children were exposed to language models that were considered meagre, restricted and grammatically incorrect. The additional punitive nature of language interactons inhibited children's ability to comprehend language (Bernstein, 1961; Gray and Klaus, 1963). Deutsch (1965) concluded that children from low socioeconomic backgrounds and minority status became less able to cope with intellectual and linguistic tasks as they moved through school. Their inability to plan verbally, maintain a sequence of thought and converse proposed barriers to academic achievement.

Typical measures of the linguistic ability of impoverished children included length of verbal response, complexity of sentence structure, proportion of parts of speech types, frequency of grammatical errors and articulation accuracy. These aspects of language typify the analytic approach to the classification of the structure of language as viewed by the formalists. Competence in language was judged in terms of correct or incorrect usage of various linguistic components be they syntactic, semantic or phonologic. Researchers adopted a highly clinical approach to the study of language structure.

The behavioural approach is best suited to evaluate responses in terms of being either correct or incorrect, occurring or non-occurring, and frequent or infrequent. Functional relationships between occurrence of responses and consequent events were analysed to determine laws of learning. These fundamental laws seemed to apply to ways in which all living organisms learned. It was apparent that behaviour could be controlled by careful manipulation of consequences. Essential to the behavioural approach is the precise definition of the response to be changed, a response capable of being increased or decreased. A behavioural approach to the treatment of delayed language seemed best suited as a means of changing language behaviour since this behaviour was considered much the same as other learned operant behaviours. Functionalists who conceived of language as a set of specific verbal behaviours needed only to apply techniques of operant conditioning to modify present language behaviours. Those responsible for the education of underprivileged, brain damaged or retarded children were especially interested in improving language abilities since numerous studies indicated poor language skills were the principal characteristic of these children (Raph, 1965).

In 1964 two educators, Bereiter and Engelmann, co-operated on joint research projects involving education of the disadvantaged child. It was their belief that traditional preschool prorgrammes offering a watered down infusion of experiences called enrichment activities were of little value to disadvantaged children. They felt radical departures from established practices of early childhood education were needed. Two years later they published an innovative book describing a curriculum guide. It included specific procedures to teach language behaviours in a step-by-step fashion (Bereiter and Engelmann, 1966). Detriments of cultural deprivation, a topic of great concern at the time, were viewed as primarily a problem of language deprivation. A major part of their book outlined a strategy for teaching language skills. It was assumed the child entered a school setting without adequate understanding of basic language concepts. The teacher's role is to demonstrate the concept by presenting examples of what the concept is and is not. The teacher then requires the child to respond, demonstrating understanding of the concept. Finally, the teacher provides feedback to the child either verifying the correct response or pointing out an error. They state (p. 123), 'The minimum teaching language must be sufficient for the two phases of the teaching presentation . . . the phase in which examples of the concept are presented, and the phase in which feedback is provided for the child'. The teaching procedure involves helping the child think logically about the environment. This is accomplished by presenting concepts such as a ball, identifying the item with the statement 'This is a ball' and asking 'Is this a ball?' or 'What is this?' Language ability is defined in terms of the child's ability to verify statements, identify concepts and describe environmental events. As the authors put it, ' . . . the basic unit of the teaching language must be the statement of fact' (p. 126). This approach to teaching language skills as defined by Bereiter and Engelmann could be taught easily using a behavioral approach where consequent events play a major role in modifying behavior. The authors state (p. 126), ' . . . the teaching of language must occur in the domain of *yes-no*'. Cookies paired with verbal praise are used as rewards for correct responses during the initial stages of treatment. Gradually, cookies are eliminated leaving verbal praise as the sole reward. Punishment is recommended as a means of decreasing incorrect responses and undesirable behaviours. At first, physical punishment is used in the form of anger, 'a slap or a good shaking' (p. 87). A loud statement 'No' is always provided following wrong responses. Isolation or time-out is also used to decrease undesired behaviour.

Thus, Bereiter and Engelmann's procedure illustrates the practical application of a straightforward behavioural approach to teaching language concepts. The modified programme, titled the 'Distar Language Program' (Engelmann, Osborn and Engelmann, 1969), is used by many teachers across the USA in place of the unstructured traditional teaching approach. The impact of this programme upon educators at the preschool and elementary levels has been substantial.

Also at this time, a number of psychologists were involved in teaching language skills to retarded and psychotic children, again using a strict behavioural approach. They, too, viewed language in terms of the formalist framework in that language could be broken down into a set of specific verbal behaviours, that is, parts of speech (nouns, verbs, etc.) that could be strung together according to certain rules to form meaningful sentences. One of the most influential books reflecting the state of the art of behavioural research in language training appeared in 1968 edited by Sloane and MacAulay. The reports included in their book represent attempts to teach speech and language skills to individual children by maintaining precise, consistent and immediate relationships between specific verbal response consequences. The rigorous control of consequences, the careful observational procedures used, and the attention given to minute details of stimulus presentation make these studies stand out as distinctly different from previous language teaching programmes. Many linguists considered their analysis of language extremely naive but few would question the rigours with which the behavioural approach was used.

One approach in Sloane and MacAulay's book clearly illustrates the use of the behavioural approach in teaching language (Risley and Wolf, 1968). In this case, the objective was to establish functional speech in children who demonstrate inappropriate verbal behaviour, chiefly echolalia. The behavioural techniques involved, shaping verbal responses through imitation of the trainer's model, the gradual introduction of new stimuli and reduction of verbal prompts to bring imitative speech responses under the control of other appropriate stimuli, and the use of differential reinforcement to increase appropriate responses and of extinction and time-out procedures to reduce inappropriate behaviours. First control over imitation was established, followed by teaching naming skills, expanding the vocabulary, evoking phrases, and finally generalising these verbal responses to the home environment. Initially, food was used as the reinforcer but gradually opportunity to obtain natural consequences was used to maintain language behaviours. For example, children learned they could control adult behaviour by using language appropriately. A child's verbal request, 'out the door' resulted in the door being opened by the adult.

Other studies reported in Sloane and MacAulay's book clearly demonstrate how the behavioural approach could be used to reinstate language in aphasic patients and in mute children and adults, to alter phonological patterns, and reduce stuttering. The research of some speech/language pathologists who were experimenting with the behavioural approach was represented (Holland and Harris, 1968; Holland and Matthews, 1968; Martin, 1968; and Mowrer, Baker and Schutz, 1968). In all cases it was demonstrated that desired responses could be increased significantly by the careful manipulation of antecedent and consequent events.

Several other studies conducted during the late 1960s with children who were deficient in verbal ability focused upon effects of different reinforcers. Reynolds and Risely (1968) used teacher attention as a consequence to increase frequency of vocalisation of a 4-year-old black girl. When this consequence was applied, rate of verbalisation increased considerably. Her use of request statements increased five-fold over nonrequest statememts. A second part of the experiment involved determining reinforcer effectiveness. It was found that teacher attention, that is, asking her what play materials she wanted, resulted in greater verbal output than did praise or social interaction. Making play materials contingent on verbalisation can be an effective way to increase speech rate.

Hart and Risley (1968) found a child's use of specific words (adjectives in this case) could be increased when play materials were contingent on the child's use of adjectives. Teacher praise and snacks were found to be ineffective reinforcers with the disadvantaged population studied.

A number of similar articles were published during the late 1960s investigating the effects of various factors upon language acquisition. One of the early attempts using operant conditioning procedures as the delivery system, but a shift in the content of the programme, was developed by Gray (1970), a speech/language pathologist. Gray viewed language as a complex system of interrelationships which represent ideas rather than a series of learned behaviours that are chained through stimulus-response bonds. His major criticism of previous attempts to teach language was their emphasis upon teaching individual verbal responses to certain classes of stimuli. He felt this approach results in the development of a surface language that lacks deep inner language structure. It is the deep structure that permits internalisation of rules and language composition resulting in the generalisation of propositional language.

Gray reasoned once we discover *which* S-R bonds must be conditioned and in what order they should be presented, propositional language could be taught. Whereas most language treatment approaches focused upon content words that have concrete lexical meanings, Gray concentrated upon teaching function words since they provided grammatical context (syntax) for the content words. He drew from the writings of Miller (1951), Bannon (1958) and Lee (1966) in organising the sequence of language learning tasks that began with a small core of content words followed by a few basic function words to form complete syntactic structures. Phonological errors, if present, were treated last. His test of language acquisition was the child's ability to generate appropriate new sentences to novel situations. The components of

Gray's programme are shown in Table 2.2.

Table 2.2: Language Components Used in Gray's Programmed Conditioning Programme (Reprinted by permission)

Area		Programme topics
Content words	1.	Common nouns and other content words
Function words	2.	is
	3.	is verb —ing
	4.	what is
	5.	is interrogative
	6.	he/she is
	7.	I am
	8.	you are
	9.	plural noun are
	10.	they are
	11.	we are
	12.	what are
	13.	are interrogative
	14.	infinitive to
	15.	comparative and superlative adjectives
	16.	regular past tense
	17.	future tense
Articulation	18.	articulation (all sounds)
Optional programmes	19.	the
	20.	who is
	21.	where is
	22.	is + negative
	23.	where are
	24.	are + negative

The conditioning part of the programme drew from behavioural models described in Wolpe (1958), Eysenck (1964), Ullman and Krasner (1966), Ulrich, Stachnik and Mabry (1966), and Wolpe and Lazarus (1966). The intent was to combine the systematic organisation and pacing of the programmed instruction with a monitoring and reward system of conditioning procedures. This Gray called 'programmed conditioning for language acquisition' (p. 104). The antecedent and consequent events were specified in terms of the stimulus to be presented, what the reponse should be, type of model used, schedule of reinforcement, criteria for advancement, stimulus and response modes, and level of stimulus complexity. The plan for presenting the 'is + ing verb' sequence is shown in Table 2.3.

Table 2.3: Delivery Design for Teaching 'is + ing verb' (Gray, 1970) (Reprinted by permission)

GOAL: Use of is verb-ing construction in spontaneous language

G: Star-token and social approval

COMMENTS: np-vp repeated twice

DATE:

	STEP	STIMULUS	RESPONSE	M	Sch	C	SM	RM	Cx
Series A	1	action np-vp	is-verb-ing	I	C	10	V/V	V	2-2
	2	action np-vp	sub-is-verb-ing	I	C	10	V/V	V	3-3
Series B	1	picture np-vp	sub-is-verb-ing	I	50	10	V/V	V	3-3
	2	picture np-vp	sub-is-verb-ing-D.O.	I	50	10	V/V	V	4-4
	3	picture np-vp	sub-is-verb-ing-D.O.	IE(art)	50	10	V/V	V	5-4
	4	picture np-vp	sub-is-verb-ing-D.O.	DE(art)	50	10	V/V	V	5-4
	5	picture np-vp	sub-is-verb-ing-D.O.	IT(sub)	50	10	V/V	V	1-4
Series C	1	picture np-vp	is-verb-ing-prep-noun	I	50	10	V/V	V	4-4
	2	picture np-vp	sub-is-verb-ing prep-noun	I	50	10	V/V	V	5-5
	3	picture np-vp	sub-is-verb-ing prep-noun	IE(art)	50	10	V/V	V	7-5
	4	picture np-vp	sub-is-verb-ing-prep-noun	DE(art)	50	10	V/V	V	7-5
	5	picture np-vp	sub-is-verb-ing-prep-noun	IT(sub)	50	10	V/V	V	1-5
Series D	1	picture non rep. question	sub-is-verb-ing-D.O./prep-noun	N	C	10	V/V	V	—
	2	picture non rep. question	sub-is-verb-ing-D.O./prep-noun	N	50	10	V/V	V	—
	3	action non rep. question	sub-is-verb-ing-D.O./prep-noun	N	I	10	V/V	V	—
	4	story-pictures non rep. question	sub-is-verb-ing-D.O./prep-noun	N	I	15	V/V	V	—
	5	spontaneous language	sub-is-verb-ing-D.O./prep-noun	N	O/social	—	O/V	C	—

Efforts were also made to generalise newly acquired language patterns from the classroom to the home environment in the following sequence: training session, show and tell, story time, juice and cookies, playground, and home. It was noted that if no effort was made to teach generalisation of new responses, they did not occur in out-of-training settings. This, Gray contended, was a major failing of most language training programmes.

Gray's work represented a significant advance in the development of a language treatment programme using a behavioural approach. His attempts to deal with content from a more sophisticated linguistic viewpoint represented a departure from previous word-building approaches. Subsequent refinements of Gray's original work were published a few years later (Gray and Ryan, 1971; Gray and Ryan, 1973).

Risely, Reynolds and Hart (1970) also realised the importance of generalisation training of language skills and developed a parent-co-operative preschool programme encompassing a behavioural approach. They noted that most parents they dealt with used inappropriate teaching strategies, that is, they rarely used positive social reinforcement and showed little understanding of how to teach complex tasks. Parents usually attempted to control behaviour with threats.

To counteract the negative aspects of parental control and assist generalisation of language usage, the authors developed a parent training programme to show mothers how to use a behavioural approach effectively. First, they trained parents to teach simple tasks to other children. A red light signalled to them when they praised the child. Rates of praise statements increased dramatically under these conditions. Nagging and aversive comments were reduced to almost zero. Then mothers were allowed to train their own children and maintained high praise rates while following highly structured teaching activities. One mother was even successul in teaching her child appropriate use of 16 consonant endings which were previously omitted.

During the early 1970s a large number of programmes were developed to teach language skills to various populations at various levels of sophistication. Most employed some form of behavioural approach, as illustrated in Table 2.4 produced by Connell (unpublished). Furthermore, Fristoe (1974) identified some 200 programmes designed to teach some aspect of language to retarded children.

In 1970, another ASHA monograph featured studies describing how operant conditioning procedures were used to alter some aspect of lan-gauge behaviour (Girardeau and Spradlin, 1970b). An outgrowth of the earlier 1963 ASHA monograph, both the result of funded research pro-

Table 2.4 List of 16 Language Programmes Available During the Late 1960s and Early 1970s (Reprinted by permission of P.J. Connell, University of Wisconsin, Madison, Wis.)

Programme	Specifically described	Content	Sequence	Entry behaviours	Exit behaviours	Training methods	Generalisation Intra	Generalisation Extra	Production and comprehension
Bricker & Bricker (1974)	No	Functional	Functional	Infants, Prelanguage	Simple sentences	Prompting & fading	+	+	Both
Carrier (1974)	Yes	Functional	Functional	Minimal language	Simple sentences	Prompting & fading	Yes	No	Both*
Dunn & Smith (1965-8)	Yes	Functional	Functional	Sophisticated language	Complex sentences	++	No	No	Both
Engelmann, Osborn & Engelmann (1969)	Yes	Functional	Functional	Some language	Simple sentences	++	Yes	No	Both
Engelmann & Osborn (1970)	Yes	Functional	Functional	Sophisticated language	Complex sentences	++	Yes	No	Both
Gray & Ryan (1971)	Yes	Syntactic	Developmental	Sophisticated language	Complex sentences	Imitation	Yes	Yes	Prod.
Guess, Sailor & Baer (1976)	+++	Functional	Functional	Minimal language	Simple sentences	Prompting & fading	Yes	Yes	Both
Kent (1974)	Yes	Functional	Functional	Minimal language	Simple sentences	Prompting & fading	Yes	Yes	Both
Lovaas (1966)	Yes	Functional	Functional	Minimal language	Simple sentences	Prompting & fading	No	No	Both
Marshall & Hegrenes (1970)	No	Functional	Functional	Some comprehension, Imitation	Simple sentences	Prompting & fading	No	No	Both+
Marshall & Hegrenes (1972)	No	Functional	Functional	Some comprehension, No production	Simple sentences	Prompting & fading	No	No	Both
Miller & Yoder (1972)	No	Syntactic & Semantic	Developmental	Some comprehension, No production	Simple sentences	Imitation, Expansion, Modelling	+	+	Both
Miller & Yoder (1974)	No	Semantic	Developmental	Verbal imitation Cognitive awareness	Two-word level	Imitation, Fading	+	+	Both
Risley & Wolfe (1968)	Yes	Functional	Functional	Echolalic behaviour	Simple sentences	Imitation, Fading	No	No	Prod.
Stremel & Waryas (1974)	No	Syntactic & Semantic	Developmental	Comprehension of commands and labels	Complex sentences	Imitation	Yes	Yes	Both
Tawney & Hipsher (1972)	Yes	Functional	Functional	Minimal language	Simple sentences	Prompting & fading	Yes	Yes	Comp.

Notes: * Nonspeech programmes
 + Programme was not described in sufficient detail to ascertain
 ++ Programmes use complex training methods which are not easily categorised.
 +++ Programme is in preparation.

jects conducted at Parsons, Kansas and the University of Kansas, the theme was to develop a systematic set of principles that could be used to devise effective procedures for changing speech behaviour. Five of the six studies used reinforcement as the principal means of increasing verbal behaviour. Time-out from reinforcement and reinforcement of incompatible behaviour were used to decelerate inappropriate behaviours. Generalisation was accomplished by shifting stimulus control to the parents in the home setting and using an intermittent reinforcement schedule. In short, speech/language pathologists were encouraged to use behavioural principles in the development of effective speech modification principles. They were also advised to design precise clinician and machine-presented instructional programmes to modify speech and language behaviours using the behavioural approach.

A behavioural approach for teaching language skills to Down's Syndrome children was advocated by Horstmeier and MacDonald (1978). Designed for parents to use in teaching their child, this programme begins by teaching motor and sound imitation, single word imitation, and two or more words in social conversation settings. Generally, parents provide stimulation, the child responds, and the child is rewarded in the typical operant conditioning format.

Psychologists who worked with retarded and autistic children have continued their study of manipulating specific language behaviours using the operant conditioning model. Guess and Baer (1973) reviewed several studies in which behavioural approaches were used to study how severely and moderately retarded children were taught grammatical rules of English morphology and generative usage of verb inflections using imitation and differential reinforcement. It was concluded that teaching a small number of exemplars in a class of linguistic behaviours generalises to other members of that response class.

McKenna-Hartung and Hartung (1973) present an extensive review of literature dealing with behavioural attempts to teach language to autistic children. They stressed the importance of selecting appropriate reinforcers, schedules of reinforcement and pairing reinforcers with verbal praise. The chief attributes of language studied by various investigators attempting to establish control over verbal responses were imitation, spontaneous naming, answering questions, establishment of phrases, conditioning functional speech and generalising appropriate speech. Finally, four studies were reviewed that reported how parents could be trained as therapists.

More recently, Essa (1978), reviewing behavioural research applied in the preschool setting, concluded the behavioural approach used in teaching language skills has been very effective. There can be no question regarding the value of these studies in identifying relevant elements of the teaching process and in applying these to demonstrate increases in specific instances of language usage. By the mid-1970s more than 200 language programmes were available, many featuring a behavioural approach. Clearly, the ten-year period between 1965 and 1975 marked the high point in using the behavioural approach to the treatment of language problems.

Current Status of the Behavioural Approach in Treating Language Problems

It should come as no surprise that the use of the behavioural approach in teaching language declined since the mid-1970s. Undoubtedly this was due to the influence of linguists who held quite different views from psychologists. Chomsky (1957, 1965) was opposed to the Skinnerian explanation of how language is learned. Chomsky viewed language acquisition as an innate recognition device (language acquisition device). The generative syntactic theories prominent during the 1960s described language in terms of a set of deep structure rules from which a child generates sentences. Gray and Ryan's (1973) programme was an attempt to utilise many of the principles of syntactic theory but used the operant paradigm as the delivery system.

Generative semantic theories emerged early in the 1970s and cast yet a different light on the acquisition of language (Slobin, 1973; Bates, 1976). The important aspect of language was the semantic knowledge the child possessed rather than syntactic knowledge. Miller and Yoder (1974) developed a language programme to teach semantic functions and used an operant conditioning framework as the teaching device.

The most recent emphasis in the study of language acquisition is in the area of pragmatics (Bruner, 1981; Gallagher and Prutting, 1983). Pragmatics is concerned with how one interacts within the social environment, not the form one uses to string words together. Important factors are eye gaze, turn-taking, communicative intentions, and sensitivity to major listener characterstics such as sex, age and status differences. Bruner (1981) feels it is the pragmatic aspects of language, not syntax structure or semantics, that mothers intuitively teach their children. Mothers spend considerable time helping their children learn how to say things that are appropriate to the situation, with less attention to grammatical form or explicit meaning. As Snow and Ferguson (1977) point out, parents play a more important role in facilitating language acquisition then merely modelling correct sentence structure or providing input for the language acquisition device.

Craig (1983), in discussing the newly emerging pragmatic language models, sees the operant conditioning paradigm as playing an important role in teaching certain language skills. Frequently, language-impaired children lack basic communicative skills that facilitate interaction with conversation partners on a pragmatic level. Clinicians skilled in using operant conditioning procedures can assist in the establishment and maintenance of critical language behaviours required to assist with peer and adult interaction. In this respect, the pathologist's responsibility is to analyse what skills are required for effective language intervention and develop procedures for presenting relevant stimuli and reinforcing events. Specialised learning situations that allow for well programmed and intensive, individualised instruction should be used when needed.

Craig also points out the pathologist must be able to serve as a language facilitator in assisting with the development of cognitive features of language. In this role, play activities are designed to provide natural contexts in which the child learns appropriate communication rules. By combining operant procedures and cognitive teaching, Craig feels we are in a much better position to teach pragmatics than using solely one method. The need lies in updating operant conditioning procedures to develop more effective techniques for teaching communicative functions.

Others see no place for using the tight control procedures so typical of operant conditioning techniques. Bruner (1981), for example, favours teaching language through the natural setting of discourse that involves the verbal interactions between a child who has a high readiness to learn the rules of the system and the expert adult, well-tuned to meet the needs of the child. The result of these interactions is, according to Bruner, a swift achievement of the syntactic, semantic and pragmatic features of language.

Neel (1983) stresses use of a natural setting to teach language to autistic children; the important element of the curriculum is to teach children to function in community settings and win the approval of significant others. Children are taught to use language behaviours in the sequence and in the environment in which they naturally occur. Thus, since the artificial and isolated clinical training programme is eliminated when a child is trained in the natural environment, there are no generalisation problems.

Neel (1983) has developed a language teaching programme for autistic children along these same pragmatic lines. He noted that while the application of behavioural technology in teaching language to autistic children clearly demonstrated autistic children could learn, the goals of these language programmes were unsound. Autistic children learned only bits and pieces of the total communication process. Whether a child knows 5 or 500 nouns makes little difference to the child who doesn't know when or where to use them. He stressed the importance of teaching functional language skills in a natural context imbedded in daily routines of the home and school using parents and teachers to deliver the programmes. The goal is to increase the autistic child's ability to control the environment using communication. It is not necessary to have an elaborate language system to communicate effectively. In many cases, gestures alone serve as adequate communication.

The language intervention programme written by Bloom and Lahey (1978) makes little mention of operant conditioning procedures. In their brief discussion of using reinforcers, they suggest the best reinforcer is to use the natural consequences of language. The response 'want cookie' should result in presentation of a cookie. They point out external forms of reinforcement should be used with caution. Starkweather (1983) commented that Bloom and Lahey take pains not to use terminology like behaviour modification in their attempt to avoid association with the highly structured operant methodology.

In reviewing current literature about teaching language skills, there seems to be a pendulum swing away from highly structured programmed tactics typical of the behavioural movement of the 1950s and 1960s. This reaction is more against the learning theory approach to language acquisition set forth by Miller and Dollard (1941), Hull (1943), Skinner (1957) and Mowrer (1960). Chomsky's (1957) criticism of Skinner's theory of language acquistion and his stress upon generative grammar followed by the emphasis upon semantic features of language and later the movement toward pragmatics has cast doubt upon the assumption that language is an operant behaviour and, as such, can be taught in the same manner as other operants.

There can be little doubt about the important advancements that have occurred during the last three decades in the area of language intervention strategies. The unfortunate thing is that many professionals responsible for devising language intervention programmes also seem to have discarded operant conditioning procedures along with the early language teaching programmes. Kanfer and Phillips (1970) make the point that behaviour modification procedures are content free; that is, no matter what theory you might be operating from, the procedures used to carry out the theory can be the same. Whether one approaches language intervention from a syntactic, semantic or pragmatic point of view, the delivery system can be similar in each case. The antecedent events are clearly marked, a target response is defined empirically, and consequences are carefully specified. Data are kept to help determine if and how rapidly behavioural change occurs and the teacher has objectives that are specified in terms of learner performance. These procedures are not incompatible with the naturalistic teaching style currently in vogue.

I am in agreement with Craig (1983) who feels we should make use of the behavioural approach in teaching language, but we need to update the methodology. Bandura's (1971) significant contribution toward understanding the role imitation and modelling play in skill acquisition represents an advance in devising more effective teaching strategies. Many aspects of his social learning theory seems to fit well with current pragmatic approaches. The issue of vicarious or observational learning discussed by Bandura and others certainly shed new light on the narrow interpretation of imititative learning theory of the 1950s.

The Behavioural Approach in Education

Although there has been a declining interest in the behavioural approach as applied to the treatment of language disorders, there continues to be strong research activity in behaviour modification procedures within the area of education. Much can be gained by keeping abreast of this research since many of the results and strategies can be applied to treating language problems.

Since reinforcement plays such an important role in operant conditioning, considerable research has been aimed at determining the most effective reinforcer for different social classes. It has been assumed that tangible reinforcers, such as candy, cookies, ice cream, toys, trinkets and money, are best suited for lower-class children who have little intrinsic motivation. Middle- and upper-class children, on the other hand, respond better to social praise and knowledge of results or even anticipation of a reward supposedly because of their advanced maturity. Russell (1971), after reviewing research pertaining to social class response to different types of reinforcement, was convinced tangible reinforcers worked best with lower-class children.

A substantial number of studies do not support the social class hypothesis as set forth by Russell and others. Schultz and Sherman (1976), reviewing some 60 studies conducted between 1966 and 1976 regarding reinforcer effectiveness and social class, concluded claims made by Russell (1971) and Spilerman (1971) regarding reinforcement preferences for lower-social class children are simply unfounded and misleading. Social class differences in reinforcer preferences cannot be assumed. Actually, the persistent use of token and tangible reinforcement for lower-class children in the long run may reduce intrinsic motivation they should derive from completing academic tasks (Levine and Fasnacht, 1974). Schultz and Sherman (1976) conclude there are no known differences in social class reinforcer preferences. Such preferences should be determined for each individual rather than by *a priori* judgement of the teacher.

Michaels (1977), in reviewing studies of reward systems used in academic set-ups, observed grades as reinforcers are effective for only the top third of the class who usually receive the highest marks. Performance gains by initially low performers are seldom reinforced, that is, followed by high grades. Michaels stressed the fact that grades, if used as a reinforcer, should be given on the basis of individual performance, not as a comparison to the performance of other individuals. Slavin (1977) also reviewed the literature pertaining to co-operative classroom reward structure. Considerable research has been conducted to determine the effect of various reward structures. Slavin concludes that co-operative reward structures in which an entire group gets rewarded for attaining some goal (most sports utilise this type) greatly increase social connectedness among students but performance is not significantly increased. Competitive and individual reward structures like grading on a curve or playing chess where one who wins necessitates one who will lose is best for increasing performance. More research is needed to discover ideal reward contingencies for maximising both student achievement and social connectedness.

Behaviour analysis research has been particularly abundant at the preschool level. Many of the findings are directly applicable to language intervention procedures, especially pragmatics. For example, most children learn the required social skills, such as how to resolve conflicts, to give and take in friendship, interact successfully with others and the like, but some children fail to acquire these social skills. For them, the goal at the preschool level is to increase peer interaction, decrease aggressive-disruptive behaviours and increase compliance and attending behaviours. Essa (1978) reviewed a number of studies designed to identify variables that affect social interaction. Reinforcement of desirable behaviour and extinction of undesirable behaviour are the most widely-used techniques used to change deviant behaviour. Modelling, a promising technique for changing behaviours, has not been utilised as much as reinforcement techniques. In dealing with aggressive-disruptive behaviours, time-out is used frequently. It was suggested that a more careful study be made of possible reinforcers, like making play materials contingent upon appropriate verbalisations. Essa concludes the behavioural approach has taken preschool education out of the realm of intuitive functioning toward a more systematic approach that will allow us to become more effective teachers.

Additional information about the use of rewards is presented by Bates (1976). After reviewing the literature dealing with extrinsic rewards and intrinsic motivation, Bates concludes we should be extremely cautious about the indiscreet use of extrinsic rewards. In his summary he concludes rewards that have been made contingent only upon participation in an activity generally result in a decreased interest in that activity, especially if it was in itself an entertaining activity. On the other hand, rewards do enhance task desirability when the task to be practiced is disliked, such as learning one's multiplication tables. But we have little information about the long-lasting effects of behavioural persistence once the rewards are removed. Another finding was that social reinforcers like praise may contribute to intrinsic motivation providing they are relevant to the task and do not occur too frequently. Social reinforcers are of greatest value in increasing behaviours that are normally not associated with tangible reinforcers.

Finally, in another review of educational research dealing with dispensing reinforcement, McGee, Kauffman and Nussen (1977) consider merits of using peers as dispensers of reinforcement. It has been well documented that peer approval for disruptive behaviours can influence acquisition and maintenance of these behaviours. Walker and Buckley (1972) utilised this strategy using peer reinforcement contingent upon desirable behaviours and were able to maintain these behaviours in this way. Children can function effectively as reinforcing agents and thus play an important part in reconstructing social environment of language-deficient children who are frequently ignored in the classroom. A number of interesting paradigms have been applied. A popular procedure is to pair two children, one as the change agent, the other as the target child. McLaughlin and Malaby (1975) summarised several studies illustrating how elementary-aged children could serve as effective behaviour observers, as teacher aides, and even as experimenters to devise and conduct behaviour change plans for other children.

In other paradigms, a group, usually a class, provides reinforcement for target behaviours. Once target behaviours have been clearly identified, peers can be observed providing encouragement, prompting and reminding to the target child. A number of variables have been investigated regarding use of peers in performance of academic tutoring. It was found that almost any child can serve as a tutor including behaviourally disoriented, mentally handicapped and learning-disabled children. Ages of tutors range from nursery school age to adolescents.

Thus we can see that a large number of innovative behavioural approaches have been introduced into the academic classroom setting to improve learning. Many of these procedures can be adapted to teaching language skills to children. Those who view operant conditioning as a situation in which candies are popped into the child's mouth after each correct response have a very narrow and distorted view of the new ways in which operant conditioning is applied in the classrooms of today.

Conclusions

Many clinicians have designed language training programmes that keep abreast of current changes in theoretical issues but continue to use the behavioural approach to deliver the programme (Bereiter and Engelmann, 1966; Gray and Ryan, 1973; Miller and Yoder, 1974; Horstmeier and MacDonald, 1978; Starkweather, 1983), while others place little or no emphasis upon the behavioural approach (Bloom and Lahey, 1978; Bruner, 1981). The predominant current attitude toward the behavioural approach in language intervention is clearly expressed in a recent article by Prizant (1982) who discusses the role of speech-language pathologists in treating autistic children. You will recall that if behavioural approaches worked well anywhere, they have proven to be very effective with autistic children. The need for a highly structured environment with consistent use of predetermined antecedent and consequent events is particularly apparent with autistic children (Donnellan-Walsh *et al.*, 1976). Yet this very structure of maintaining set routines eventually becomes a hindrance and sometimes presents obstacles to learning new skills (Shepard and Shepard, 1980). The focus of language intervention programmes today is upon adaptability and flexibility not specified repertoires of verbal behaviours usually taught using behavioural approaches. The major criticism of behavioural approaches is that they focus upon teaching children to respond correctly rather than to be an initiator of communication. As Caparulo and Cohen (1977) put it (p. 622), 'We have become increasingly suspicious of results of standard laboratory set-up, which may provide the control of variables but fail to reveal how closely performance is connected to functioning of motivation state, at any particular moment'. Prizant (1982) feels that behavioural approaches have failed to take into account important variables like motivational states and cognitive features. These variables are ignored by behaviourists because they can't be measured. Neel (1983) also stresses the fact that we need to take into account features other than just those that can be objectively measured if we are to experience success in treating autistic children. This failure to consider unobservable events is a major criticism of the behavioural approach.

Research activity involving the use of operant conditioning is much more active in classroom settings where academics are taught. An important lesson to be learned from this research is that there is much more to be known about the effective use of operant conditioning procedures than we suspected back in the 1960s. I think it is unfortunate that presently there is so little research activity in the area of the behavioural approach to language learning. There is a strong tendency to associate simplistic language learning theory with the operant conditioning procedures, negating both in the process. What is needed is continued research activity to help us find more effective ways of manipulating language behaviour through behavioural approaches. We have much to gain by keeping abreast of current behavioural research classroom learning situations.

References

Addison, R.M. and Homme, L.E. (1966) The reinforcing event (re) menu, *National Society for Programmed Instruction Journal, 5*, 8-9

Ayllon, T. and Azrin, N.H. (1968) *The Token Economy: A Motivational System For Therapy and Rehabilitation*, Appleton-Century-Crofts, New York

Baer, D.M. and Wolf, M.M. (1968) The reinforcement contingency in preschool and remedial education, in R.D. Hess and D.M. Baer (eds.), *Early Childhood Education*, Aldine, Chicago

Bandura, A. (1971) *Psychological Modeling; Conflicting Theories*, Aldine, Chicago

Bannon, J.B. (1958) Linguistic word classes in the spoken language of normal, hard-of-hearing, and deaf children, *Journal of Speech and Hearing Research*, *11*, 279-87

Bates, E. (1976) Pragmatics and sociolinguistics in child language, in D. Morehead and A. Morehead (eds.), *Language Deficiency in Children: Selected Readings*, University Park Press, Baltimore.

Bereiter, C. and Engelmann, S. (1966) *Teaching Disadvantaged Children in The Preschool*, Prentice Hall, Engelwood Cliffs, New Jersey

Bernstein, B. (1961) Social class and linguistic development; a theory of social learning, in A.H. Halsey, J. Floud and C.A. Anderson (eds.), *Education, Economy And Society*, Free Press of Glencoe, New York

Bijou, S.W. (1970) What psychology has to offer education – now, *Journal of Applied Behavioral Analysis*, *3*, 65-71

Birnbrauer, J.S., Burchard, J.D. and Burchard, S.N. (1970) Wanted: behavior analysis, in R.H. Bradfield (ed.), *Behavior Modification: The Human Effort*, Dimensions Pub. Co., San Rafael, California

Bloom, L. and Lahey, M. (1978) *Language Development and Language Disorders*, John Wiley and Sons, New York

Brodbeck, A.J. and Irwin, O.C. (1946) The speech behavior of infants without families, *Child Development*, *17*, 145-56

Brookshire, R.H. (1967) Speech pathology and the experimental analysis of behavior, *Journal of Speech and Hearing Disorders*, *32*, 215-27

Brown, F. (1944) An experimental and critical study of the intelligence of negro and white kindergarten children, *Journal of Genetic Psychology*, *65*, 161-75

Bruner, J. (1981) The social context of language, *Language and Communication*, *I*, 155-78

Caparulo, B. and Cohen, D. (1977) Cognitive structures, language and emerging social competence in autistic and aphasic children, *Journal of Child Psychiatry*, *15*, 620-44

Chomsky, N. (1957) *Syntactic Structures*, Mouton, The Hague
——(1965) *Aspects of the Theory of Syntax*, MIT Press, Cambridge

Craig, H.K. (1983) Applications of pragmatic language models for intervention, in M.T. Gallagher and C.A. Prutting (eds.), *Pragmatic Assessment and Intervention Issues in Language*, College-Hill Press, San Diego, California

Davis, E.A. (1937) The development of linguistic skill in twins, singletons with siblings and only children from age five to ten years, *Institute of Child Welfare Monograph Series No. 14*, University of Minnesota Press, Minneapolis

Day, E.J. (1932) The development of language in twins: I. a comparison of twins and single children, *Child Development*, *3*, 179-99

Deutsch, M. (1965) The role of social class in language development and cognition, *American Journal of Orthopsychiatry*, *35*, 78-88

Donnellan-Walsh, A., Gossage, L.D., La Vigna, G.W., Schuler, A.L. and Traphagen, J.D. (1976) *Teaching Makes the Difference*, State Dept. of Education, Sacramento, California

Engelmann, S., Osborn, J. and Engelmann, T. (1969) *Distar Language I, Teacher's Guide*, Science Research Associates, Chicago

Essa, E.L. (1978) The preschool: setting for applied behavior analysis, *Review of Educational Research*, *48*, 537-75

Eysenck, H.J. (1964) *Experiments in Behavior Therapy*, Pergamon, London

Fleming, V.V.D. (1942) A study of Stanford-Binet vocabulary attainment and growth in chidren in the City of Childhood, Mooseheart, Illinois, as compared with children living in their own homes, *Journal of Genetic Psychology*, *60*, 359-73

Fowler, W. (1962) Cognitive learning in infancy and early childhood, *Psychological Bulletin*, *59*, 116-52

Fristoe, M. (1974) *Language Intervention System for the Retarded: A Catalogue of Original Language Structured Programs in the U.S.*, State of Alabama Dept. of Education, Montgomery, Alabama

Gallagher, M.T. and Prutting, C. (1983), *Pragmatic Assessment and Intervention Issues in Language*, College-Hill Press, San Diego, California

Girardeau, F.L. and Spradlin, J.E. (1970a) An introduction to the functional analysis of speech and language, in F.L. Girardeau and J.E. Spradlin (eds.), *A Functional Analysis Approach to Speech and Language, ASHA Monographs, 14*, ASHA, Washington, 1-9

——and Spradlin, J.E. (1970b) *A Functional Analysis Approach To Speech and Language, ASHA Monographs, 14*, ASHA, Washington

Goldfarb, W. (1945) Effects of psychological deprivation in infancy and subsequent stimulation, *American Journal of Psychiatry, 102*, 18-33

Gray, B.B. (1970) Language acquisition through programmed conditioning, in R.H. Bradfield (ed.), *Behavior Modification: The Human Effort*, Dimensions Pub. Co., San Rafael, California

——and Ryan, B.A. (1971) *Programmed Conditioning for Language: Program Book*, Monterey Learning Systems, Monterey, California

——and Ryan, B.A. (1973) *A Language Program For The Nonlanguage Child*, Research Press, Champaign, Illinois

Gray, S. and Klaus, R. (1963) *Early Training Project: Interim Report*, The City Schools and George Peabody College for Teachers, Murfreesboro, TN (mimeo)

Grings, W.W. and Carlin, S. (1966) Instrumental modification of autonomic behavior, *Psychological Record, 16*, 153-9

Guess, D. and Baer, D.M. (1973) Some experimental analyses of linguistic development in institutionalized retarded children, in B.B. Lahey (ed.), *The Modification of Language Behavior*, Charles C. Thomas, Springfield, Illinois

Hanley, E.M. (1970) Review of research involving applied behaviors in the classroom, *Review of Educational Research, 40*, 597-628

Hart, B. and Risley, T.R., (1968) Establishing the use of descriptive adjectives in the spontaneous speech of disadvantaged preschool children, *Journal of Applied Behavior Analysis, 1*, 109-20

Helmer, J.E. and Furedy, J.J. (1968) Operant conditioning of GSR amplitude, *Journal of Experimental Psychology, 78*, 463-7

Holland, A. (1967) Some application of behavioral principles to clinical speech problems, *Journal of Speech and Hearing Disorders, 32*, 11-18

——and Harris, A. (1968) Aphasia rehabilitation using programmed instruction: an intensive case history, in H. Sloane and B. MacAulay (eds.), *Operant Procedures in Remedial Speech and Language Training*, Houghton Mifflin, Boston

—— and Matthews, J. (1968) Application of teaching machine concepts to speech pathology and audiology, in H. Sloane and B. MacAulay (eds.), *Operant Procedures in Remedial Speech and Language Training*, Houghton Mifflin, Boston

Horstmeier, D.S. and MacDonald, J.D. (1978), *Ready, Set, Go: Talk To Me*, Charles Merrill, Columbus, Ohio

Hull, C.L. (1943) *Principles of Behavior*, Appleton-Century-Crofts, New York

Hunt, J. McV. (1961) *Intelligence and Experience*, Ronald Press, New York

Johnston, M. and Harris, F.R. (1968) Observation and recording of verbal behavior in remedial speechwork, in H. Sloane and B. MacAulay (eds.), *Operant Procedures in Remedial Speech and Language Training*, Houghton Mifflin, New York

Kanfer, F.H. and Phillips, J.S. (1970) *Learning Foundations of Behavior Therapy*, John Wiley and Sons, New York

Lee, L.L. (1966) Developmental sentence types, a method for comparing normal and deviant syntactic development, *Journal of Speech and Hearing Disorders*,

31, 311-30

Levine, F.M. and Fasnacht, G. (1974) Token rewards may lead to token learning, *American Psychologist, 29*, 816-20

Lindsley, O.R. (1964) Direct measurement and prosthesis of retarded behavior, *Journal of Education, 147*, 62-81

Lovaas, O.I. (1968) A program for the establishment of speech in psychotic children, in H. Sloane and B. MacAulay (eds.), *Operant Procedures in Remedial Speech and Language Training*, Houghton Mifflin, Boston

Martin, R. (1968) The experimental manipulation of stuttering behaviors, in H. Sloane and B. MacAulay (eds.), *Operant Procedures in Remedial Speech and Language Training*, Houghton Mifflin, Boston

McCarthy, D.A. (1930) The language development of the preschool child, *Institute of Child Welfare Monograph No. 4*, University of Minnesota Press, Minneapolis

McGee, C.S., Kauffman, J.M. and Nussen, J.L. (1977) Children as therapeutic change agents: reinforcement intervention paradigms, *Review of Educational Research, 47*, 451-77

McKenna-Hartung, S. and Hartung, J.R. (1973) Establishing verbal imitation skills and functional speech in autistic children, in B.B. Lahey (ed.), *The Modification of Language Behavior*, Charles C. Thomas, Springfield

McLaughlin, T.F. and Malaby, J.E. (1975) Elementary school children as behavioral engineers, in E. Ramp and G. Semb (eds.), *Behavior Analyses: Areas of Research and Application*, Prentice-Hall, Englewood Cliffs, New Jersey

McReynolds, L. (1970) Contingencies and consequences in speech therapy, *Journal of Speech and Hearing Disorders, 35*, 12-24

——and Huston (1970) Token loss in speech imitation training, *Journal of Speech and Hearing Disorders, 36*, 486-95

Michaels, J.W. (1977) Classroom reward structures and academic performance, *Review of Educational Research, 47*, 87-98

Miller, G. (1951) *Language and Communication*, McGraw Hill, New Jersey

Miller, J. and Yoder, D. (1974) An ontogenetic language teaching strategy for retarded chldrren, in R. Schiefelbush and L. Lloyd (eds.), *Language Perspectives — Acquisition, Retardation, and Intervention*, University Park Press, Baltimore

Miller, N.E. and Dollard J.(1941) *Social Learning and Imitation*, Yale University Press, New Haven

Mowrer, D.E., Baker, B.L. and Schutz, R.E. (1968) Operant procedures in the control of speech articulation, in H. Sloane and B. MacAulay (eds.), *Operant Procedures in Remedial Speech and Language Training*, Houghton Mifflin, Boston

Mowrer, O.H. (1960) *Learning Theory and Behavior*, John Wiley and Sons, New York

Neel, R.S. (1983) *Innovative Model Program For Autistic Children And Their Teachers*, unpublished manuscript, University of Washington, Seattle

Pasamanick, B. (1946) A comparative study of behavioral development of negro infants, *Journal Of Genetic Psychology, 69*, 3-44

Pierrel, R. and Sherman, J.G. (1963) Train your pet the Barnabus way, *Brown Alumni Monthly*, February, 8-14

Prizant, B.M. (1982) Speech-language pathologists and autistic children: What is our role? *ASHA, 24*, 531-6

Rachlin, H. (1970) *Introduction to Modern Behaviorism*, W.H. Freeman, San Francisco

Raph, J.B. (1965) Language development in socially disadvantaged children. *Review of Education Research, 35*, 389-400

Rescorla, R.A. and Solomon, R.L. (1967) Two-process learning theory: Relationships between Pavolovian conditioning and instrumental learning, *Psychological Review, 74*, 151-82

Reynolds, N.J. and Risely, T.R. (1968) The role of social and material reinforcers, in increasing talking of a disadvantaged preschool child, *Journal of Applied Behavior Analysis, 1*, 253-62

Risley, T. and Baer, D. (1973) Operant behavior modification: the deliberate development of behavior, in B.M. Caldwell and H.M. Ricciuti, (eds.), *Review of Child Development Research, Volume 3*, University of Chicago Press, Chicago
——Reynolds, N. and Hart, B. (1970) Behavior modification with disadvantaged preschool children, in R.H. Bradfield (ed.), *Behavior Modification: The Human Effort*, Dimensions Pub. Co., San Rafael, California
——and Wolf, M. (1968) Establishing functional speech in echolalic children, in H. Sloane and B. MacAulay (eds.), *Operant Procedures in Remedial Speech and Language Training*, Houghton Mifflin, Boston

Russell, I.L. (1971) *Motivation*, W.C. Brown, Dubuque, Iowa

Shiefelbusch, R.L. (1963) Introduction, *Journal of Speech and Hearing Disorders, Monograph Supplement 10*, ASHA, Washington, 3-8

Schultz, C.B. and Sherman, R.H. (1976) Social Class development and differences in reinforcer effectiveness, *Review of Educational Research, 46*, 25-51

Shelton, R.L. Jr., Arndt, W.B. Jr. and Miller, J.B. (1961) Learning principles and teaching of speech and language, *Journal of Speech and Hearing Disorders, 4*, 368-76

Shepard, T. and Shepard, W. (1980), Parents Viewpoint: Living with a child who has autistic tendencies, Paper presented at the Southern Illinois Second Annual Conference on Communicative Disorders, May

Sherman, J.A. (1965) Use of reinforcement and imitation to reinstate verbal behavior in mute psychotics, *Journal of Abnormal Psychology, 70*, 155-64

Sidman, M. (1965) *The Lavers Hall Project*, mimeograph, June

Skinner, B.F. (1957) *Verbal Behavior*, Appleton-Century-Crofts, New York
—— (1966) A case history in scientific method, in R.A. King (ed.), *Readings for an Introduction to Psychology* (2nd ed.), McGraw-Hill, New York

Slavin, R.E. (1977) Classroom reward structure: An analytical and practical review, *Review of Educational Research, 47*, 633-50

Sloane, H. and MacAulay, B. (1968) *Operant Procedures in Remedial Speech and Language Training*, Houghton Mifflin, Boston

Slobin, D.I. (1973) Cognitive pre-requisites for the acquisition of grammar, in C.A. Ferguson and D.I. Sobin (eds.), *Studies of Child Language and Development*, Holt, Rinehart and Winston, New York

Snow, C.E. and Ferguson, C.A. (1977) *Talking to Children: Language Input and Acquisition*, Cambridge University Press, Cambridge

Spilerman, S. (1971) Raising academic motivation in lower class adolescents: A convergence of two research traditions, *Sociology and Education, 44*, 103-18

Starkweather, C.W. (1983) *Speech and Language: Principles and Processes of Behavioral Change*, Prentice-Hall, Englewood Cliffs, New Jersey

Ullman, L.P. and Krasner, L. (1966) (eds.), *Case Studies in Behavior Modification*, Holt, Rinehart and Winston, New York

Ulrich, R., Stachnik, T. and Mabry, J. (1966) *Control of Human Behavior*, Scott, Foreman and Co., Glenview, Illinois

Walker, H.M. and Buckley, M.K. (1972) Programming generalization and maintenance of teatment effects across time and across settings, *Journal of Applied Behavior Analysis, 5*, 209-24

Wolpe, J. (1958) *Psychotherapy by Reciprocal Inhibition*, Stanford University Press, Palo Alto, California
—— and Lazarus, A. (1966) *Behaviour Therapy Techniques*, Pergamon Press, Oxford

3 RECENT DEVELOPMENTS IN PRAGMATICS: REMEDIAL IMPLICATIONS

James McLean and Lee K. Snyder-McLean

In 1927, behavioural psychologist Grace DeLaguna wrote the following:

> Once we deliberately ask the question: — *What does speech do? What objective function does it perform in human life?* — the answer is not far to seek. Speech is the great medium through which human cooperation is brought about. It is the means by which the diverse activities of men are coordinated and correlated with each other for the attainment of reciprocal ends. Men do not speak simply to relieve their feelings or to air their views, but to awaken a response in their fellows and to influence their attitudes and acts. (DeLaguna, 1963, pp. 19-20, first published in 1927.)

This need to influence the attitudes and acts of other people is now seen as exerting profound influence on the language behaviours of both children and adults. There is robust empirical evidence that behaviours designed to influence other people begin in early infancy, long before language is acquired (Bates, Camaioni and Volterra, 1975; Mahoney, 1975; Bates, 1976). There is further evidence that after language is acquired, many aspects of its *content* and *grammatical form* are shaped by this ultimate function of language as a social tool to act on others. Yet, for nearly 50 years following DeLaguna's observations, the most dominant theories of language moved further and further away from the consideration of language in the context of its human users and its human uses. While a view of language as a social tool remained at least intuitively ingrained in theorists, researchers and child-workers in remedial language, their primary attention remained focused on the *medium* of this social function — the behaviours and systems of language itself. As a result, attention to the sound systems, vocabulary and grammar systems of human language has dominated the literature of the past 30 or more years (cf. Bar-Adon and Leopold, 1971).

The peak of this attention to language behaviours and the 'rules' that controlled them, was attained in the 1950s and early 1960s when theoretical linguists and behavioural psychologist fleshed-out and firmed-up their disparate, but curiously complementary, views of human language. The complementary nature of these two antagonistic views stems from the fact that both of them were clearly focused on the explanation of language behaviours in ways that obviated the need to consider the influence of any *specific* user or use of these behaviours. Consider that Chomsky's (1957, 1965) model of transformational grammar not only ignored the potential meaning of any grammar form, but, through its 'innateness hypothesis', removed any consideration of a constructive process for language acquisition by its human users. Similarly, although Skinner's (1957) model for 'verbal behaviour' would seem to reflect a strong consideration of the functions of language, it required that only 'observable' stimuli be considered in the identification of such functions. This requirement precluded the consideration of many of the complex internal and external social variables that are now considered to characterise natural communicative language use. Thus clinical applications of Skinner's model have generally been characterised by the use of highly synthetic antecedent stimuli (e.g. a picture and the question, "What is this?") as well as the use of highly arbitrary consequent stimuli (e.g. an "M&M" candy and the phrase, "good talking"). While such stimuli are observable, they seem clearly to under-represent many of the social variables that function to control actual language use.

Even while recognising their limitations, we must also appreciate the contributions that both theoretical linguistics and operational behaviourism have brought to the treatment of deficient language systems and communicative behaviours. The linguistic models emphasise the demands that are inherent in attaining language structures that are meaningful to members of various language communities. The behavioural models and the empirical data which have been generated in their applications, emphasise that language behaviours can be modified by external arrangements of both antecedent and consequent variables. What does seem necessary now, however, is an awareness that both the linguistic and the behavioural models *under-represent* some factors of human language and human language *use* which are critical to a complete model of this important domain. Particularly, the relative failures of linguistics and behaviourism would seem to emphasise that the operationalisation of idealised, reductionistic models is not adequate either fully to describe communicative repertoires or to direct the design of remedial programmes aimed at their modification.

Obviously, it is not appropriate simply to reject the adequacy of past models. Rather, revised models must be developed which both improve and extend past models. In order to begin this process, it will help us to look carefully at the details of human language use and identify the variables in this process which appear necessary and important to a revised model. The source of theory and empirical data in this general area is found in the study of *pragmatics*.

Pragmatics and its Dimensions

Attempts to define pragmatics usually begin with the work of Morris (1946) who differentiated three dimensions of the study of language. Morris defined *pragmatics* as the study of the relations of 'signs' to their human users, as compared to *semantics* which is the study of the relations of signs to their referents and *syntactics* which is the study of the relations of signs to other signs. Such a definition, however, contributes only minimally to an appreciation of the scope of this area or the richness of the concepts and empirical findings it has generated. In order to foster these latter appreciations, we shall begin with some broad indications of what this field of study provides.

(i) Pragmatics directs us to consider the details of the *social-functions* of language, for example what specific effects is language employed to have on our fellow humans?

(ii) Pragmatics directs us to consider the influences that a speaker's *communicative history with a receiver* and the specific *physical context* of their communicative exchange have on the content and form of language utterances.

(iii) Pragmatics directs us to consider the influences that a particular *speaker's social relationship to a receiver* has on the content and form of the language employed in a communicative exchange.

(iv) Pragmatics directs us to consider the effects that a culture's *rules* for communicative exchange have on the content and form of utterances.

Even when presented at such *macro* levels, the significance of these potential contributions of pragmatics to remedial programming should be rather obvious. When each of these dimensions is fleshed-out in all of its detail, the profound level of their impact on both theory and educational application should take on even more obvious significance to the remedial language professional. To that end, we shall now endeavour to look at the detail of each of the dimensions identified above. Within these expositions, we shall also begin to anticipate some of the implications each of these dimensions has for remedial programme designs and procedures.

The Social Functions of Language Behaviours

Probably the most basic element of the study of pragmatics is the underlying assumption that human communicative behaviours carry a specific intent to, as DeLaguna (1963, pp. 19-20) stated, '. . . awaken a response in their fellows and influence their attitudes and acts'. Such an intent, DeLaguna suggests, is necessary in order that human animals co-ordinate their activities and establish the co-operative routines that enable the overall maintenance of their environments. If we consider the fact that the modern world is now fully socialised in the sense that human work, pleasure and protection are all attained in co-operative interactions with our 'fellows', the importance of this ability would be difficult to overemphasise.

In the face of this essential need to affect one another, it should not be too surprising to find that the means to this end are well developed in the human animal. This need to affect others provides considerable motivation for, and influence on, the behaviours of our children; and the training of children to have these social effects dominates our child-rearing practices. Thus the study of communication and language would seem profitably begun by looking at their most primitive forms in infants and tracing their eventual representation in the linguistic responses of children and adults. This ontogenic approach will also set the stage for our application of this area of knowledge to severely handicapped children who come to us with no linguistic responses.

Early Communicative Effects. The research of Bates and her colleagues (Bates *et al.*, 1975; Bates, 1976; Bates, 1979) provides a particularly rich exposition of the emergence and eventual differentiation of infant behaviours which seem to represent the roots of intentional communicative behaviours. In this research, Bates and her colleagues note that behaviours that have communicative effects on caregivers are present even before infants understand this ability. For example, very young infants will smile, reflexively grasp a finger placed in their palm, and will orient toward changes in their visual and auditory environment. Infants will also produce some reflexive vocal noises like sighs, gurgles and squeals. All of these vocal and nonvocal behaviours are carefully observed by caregivers and, with unerring consistency, are 'read' by these caregivers for any cues that might provide as to the infant's particular state of comfort or need. In a sense, these purely reflexive signals are assigned communicative significance by adults. Bates (1976) notes that these behaviours are obviously not 'intentional' communicative acts on the part of the infant, but, most often, caregivers treat them as though they were. Upon hearing a particular insistent cry, mothers will often respond to an infant with some rhetorical utterances like, 'Oh, is something wrong? I'll bet you're hungry aren't you? Well, mummy has a bottle warming, okay?'

Such 'assigning of intent' to infant behaviours continues into later periods of infancy where children's behaviours are no longer just reflexive, but are at levels which clearly reflect some intent or purpose — but at which they presumably do not yet understand that their behaviours can be used specifically to direct the behaviours of others. For example, a young child of seven or eight months may be reaching for a favourite toy which is beyond reach and find the toy immediately proferred by a mother saying, 'Want your Teddy? Here it is!' Almost all purposeful motor acts by infants can be (and often are) assigned communicative 'meaning' by attentive mothers and other family caregivers, yet, it is intuitively clear to these caregivers that the infant had not actually intended to affect their behaviours. Bates *et al.* (1975) call these early behaviours 'sensori-motor performatives' and note that the attention of infants in this state is narrowly focused on the object of their reach or manipulation and do not, at this point, include attention to the caregiver as a possible receiver of a behavioural 'message'.

Intentional Communication. In normally developing infants between nine and twelve months, however, Bates *et al.* (1975) observed a change in their efforts to obtain an object, make some toy perform, or protest the loss of a possession to a sibling. During this period, young children would not only carry out their normal motor responses, but would also begin to shift their gaze to the caregiver and, perhaps, add some intonated vocalisation. The fact that these episodes of 'dual regard' to both the goal of their actions and to the caregiver were consistent and persisted until the caregiver responded with appropriate help or remedy, prompted Bates and her colleagues to conclude that this particular repertoire signalled 'communicative intention' on the part of the infant, that is the infant intended these behaviours to have a specific effect on the behaviour of another person. Along with these appeals for helpful actions, Bates and her colleagues noted that their subjects' repertoires also began to include similar dual-regard repertoires to direct caregivers' attention to objects or events at times when no clear response was indicated other than the desire for the caregiver to *attend* to the object or event. Bates *et al.* (1975) differentiated these two non-verbal repertoires as *proto-imperatives* and *proto-declaratives* in order to mark their prototypic representation of later linguistic forms which have analogous differential intents.

These initial and primitive action schemes of dual regard, intonated vocalisations and sensori-motor schemes on objects have been observed to be rather quickly supplemented by additional, more refined, communicative motor acts. A natural 'gestural complex' (Bates *et al.*, 1975) is added to children's repertoires and includes: a request gesture; a give gesture; a show gesture; and a pointing (indicating) gesture. These gestures, when produced in combination with an appropriately intonated vocalisation and perhaps a visual regard of an intended referent, allow young children to carry out the relatively rich array of communicative functions shown in Table 3.1.

Table 3.1: Proto-performative Classes

Type	Definition
Proto-imperatives (consumable-food or drink)	Child directs receiver's attention to consumable item and/or uses reach gesture; is dissatisfied if adult only comments on item — clearly is requesting item
Proto-imperative (non-food-related objects, persons, actions)	Same as above, but referent item is a non-consumable object, person, or *action*
Proto-declarative	Child uses gestures (point or show) and visual regard to direct receiver's attention to an entity or event of interest — is satisfied by some comment by adult — does not seem to be requesting object
Proto-interrogative	Child directs receiver's attention to referent of interest and produces vocalisation with rising intonation — looks to adult for some answer response
Answer or reply (nonverbal)	Child responds to another's utterance with a gesture or action which serves as a relevant answer or response to the other's utterance
Greeting	Child waves and/or vocalises to signal awareness of the arrival or departure of another person. (May be cued by a similar gesture/vocalisation from the other.)

Source: Bates, *et al.*, 1975; Dore, 1975; McLean, Snyder-McLean and Cirrin, 1981; McLean *et al.*, 1982, with permission.

Along with the refinement of these gestural systems, young children also begin to refine and focus their vocal behaviours. In this process, certain sounds and sound combinations begin to be used consistently to mark certain intents or functions. These proto-words soon perform a relatively full range of instrumental and directive functions aimed at the behaviours of their caregivers. They also begin to reflect the referencing function in which they 'stand for' objects and actions in the child's world (Bates, Benigni, Bretherton, Camaioni, and Volterra, 1977; Halliday, 1975). From these proto-words, children move into conventional words and, then, progress on into multi-word utterances.

As children move into multi-word linguistic structures, the functions of their communicative acts remain of the same *genre* as those observed in the prelinguistic stages. Table 3.2 shows one taxonomy that can be applied to communicative acts which have attained linguistic levels.

Table 3.2: Communicative Intents Expressed in Early Child Language

Initiated by child in a communicative context	*Greet* (I) *Regulate* listener's attention: — to self — to referent of interest *Regulate* listener's action: — to obtain specified reinforcer — to engage in interaction *Request* information from listener
Produced by child as response to other's utterance in a dialogue context	Repeat/Imitate Greet (II) Answer Reply Continuant
Uttered in non-communicative context	Label (referential) Rehearse/Word play (non-referential)

Sources: Bruner (1975); Dore (1975); Halliday (1975); Owens (1978); McLean *et al.*, 1982, with permission.

The orderly and rather relentless movement of normally developing infants and young children from primitive motor schemes to highly conventionalised motor gestural systems and from reflexive vocalisations and, thence, into proto-words and true words in just over a year's time is truly a wonderous thing. The fact that the later appearing linguistic forms appear to 'map on to' already existing motor and vocal repertoires and the communicative functions already carried by these more primitive, nonverbal forms provides a strong rationale for viewing language behaviours in terms of their socio-communicative functions as well as their more formal linguistic forms. It seems abundantly clear that the products of the language learning process include learning how to *do things* with language as well as learning the forms of language itself.

Such a functional perspective on the *products* of language acquisition integrates well with the current notion that specific and consistent social processes appear to provide the contexts and the independent variables that are crucial to language learning. Bruner (1975) focused attention on the mother-child dyad as an interactive social context committed to the attainment of 'joint action routines' which, in their turn, required the attainment of 'joint attention' among these mothers and their young children. Bruner noted that such contexts provided both the need for, and the reward of, communicative repertoires to direct the behaviours of others and to establish attention to either one of them, or to some other object or action in the environment. Such functions are, of course, the basic imperative and declarative functions observed by Bates *et al.* (1975) in the earliest communicative acts of young infants of eight or nine months of age. As such adult-caregiver routines are continued into childhood, it is clear that the full range of proto-performatives (Table 3.1) and performatives (Table 3.2) become both needed and rewarded. Thus Bruner (1975) suggested that language form was acquired in the *service* of communicative functions, a view which was essentially at odds with both the linguist's view of the primacy of language form rules in the determination of utterances, and the behaviourist's emphasis on objective stimuli as the controlling element of utterance form. This socio-communicative perspective is widely prevalent today as remedial designers seek to teach communicative forms in the 'natural' contexts of their actual functions to affect other people in socially interactive situations. Such an approach is in dramatic contrast with those programmes which concentrate on teaching linguistic forms, or those programmes which teach linguistic forms under the control of synthetic stimuli like pictures or imitative models reinforced by arbitrary consequences like edibles or tokens.

In addition to their important implications for designing the social contexts for remedial language programming, these data on the functions of communicative behaviours offer other extremely important directions for remedial programmes. In their tracking of the emergence of various types and levels of responses which are clearly intended to have effects on the behaviours of others, researchers in pragmatics have also provided the bases for considering communicative response topographies below the level of linguistic forms. Traditional remedial language programmes have targeted both the speech mode and the linguistic response form. In fact, behaviourists have suggested that no prerequisites to these response levels can be identified and, thus, nothing below these should be considered (Guess, Sailor and Baer, 1977). Obviously, linguists do not concern themseves with communicative responses below the level of linguistic form. The developmental data on the emergence of prelinguistic communicative forms and functions, however, suggest that programmes might be directed to gestural levels or even more primitive form levels with children demonstrating severe communicative deficits. Clearly, the intent here would not be to deny speech or linguistic forms to children, but, rather, to be able to offer somewhat 'natural' and somewhat conventionalised communicative responses to children who do not show either the motor or cognitive skills needed for speech or complex symbolic structures.

The overall effects of research on the performative functions of language, then, are three-dimensional. First, they point to truly social interactive contexts for teaching and learning of communication and language. Second, they offer a broad range of communicative functions which can guide language programmes. Language, obviously, does not just 'name things'; it requests things, it asks, it directs listeners' attention, and it answers the queries of others. Third, the data in this domain identify a continuum of functional, conventionalised response levels below the level of linguistic structure which might serve as highly useful targets among children for whom linguistic forms might have a low probability at the time remedial programming is begun.

Influence of Physical Contexts and the Speaker's Communicative History

Previous models of language which have concentrated on either linguistic rules or objective stimulus control as determiners of content not only ignore the absolute functions of human communication, but they also ignore the influence that the context of an utterance and a speaker's history with a listener have on utterance selection and contruction. If we consider a communicative exchange like the following, we can see both of these at work:

'Give me the book.'
'Which one?'
'The one you were talking about.'
'Where is it?'
'On the big table — next to the ashtray.'

In this utterance, both the physical context of the exchange and the past communicative exchange of the listener and speaker contribute to the particular propositions and constructions of the utterances used.

Bates (1976) calls the mechanisms at work here 'psychological presuppositions', quite a straightforward term in this context in that they mark the elements of the physical setting and past conversations that might be assumed in a speaker's construction of a particular utterance. Consideration of these mechanisms has great potential for helping return language to its users, because they offer an alternative to the synthetic and idealised utterance structures suggested by reductionistic models. So often, the idealised models have led us to teach an utterance like, 'The boy is sleeping in his bed' and then to find ourselves wondering why this structure, so carefully modelled and reinforced to a picture stimulus, doesn't generalise to 'natural' settings. In reality, it is almost impossible to identify a 'natural' context in which such an utterance would be used (or be useful). In a very real sense, clinicians have substituted their own psychological processes for those of their language-impaired clients.

Concentration on a child's perceptions of the world, on a child's unique history with a listener, and the specific communicative context would radically alter our programming goals. It would allow us to let children talk about things in terms of their own psychological reality rather than the supposed controls structured by synthetic models. Although children's 'presuppositions' are not the same as those of a mature adult speaker, it is clear that they make them. For example, a child might look at a picture of a horse and utter, 'Grandmamma's' thus marking the place where he or she saw a horse. Clinicians are forever experiencing the mis-match between a child's 'referencing strategies' (McLean and Snyder-McLean, 1978) and their own. Too often, the child's is rejected and the clinician's prevails. It is not merely the unsatisfying exchange that is a problem here. The more important factor is that remedial programmes must begin to reflect an awareness that language is *not* adequately represented by a series of idealised syntactic structures to be modelled and acquired. Rather, language is a system which can be used to *externalise* the internal schemas and strategies of child speakers, in the context of their use, to communicate with other people toward some purpose (Olson, 1970). To be sure, appropriate grammatical structures must be used to ensure effective and efficient communication, but such structures can be taught to encode *child* meaning just as well as it can be taught to encode idealised, adult meanings.

Again, the remedial implications of this dimension of pragmatics appear to be both obvious and powerful. If our child clients are to attain language forms that are useful to them then we must target those forms which belong to them and those which encode their perceptions of the world and their communicative strategies and goals. The data on natural language learning by young children show that caregivers intuitively recognise this need to preserve child perspectives in the teaching of appropriate language structures. These data show that the natural strategy for attaining this goal is to amend and emend child utterances in ways that preserve the meanings and functions intended by the child, and to do so in the immediate context of the child's focus and communicative intentions (Moerk, 1977; Snyder-McLean and McLean, 1978).

Clearly, these perspectives are but another strong contribution to the notion that remedial programmes should be carried out in the contexts of actual language use so that targeted responses reflect both the current context of an utterance and the previous communicative history with a listener. These perspectives allow clinicians to target appropriate pronominalisation and enable them to accept normal ellipses in child utterances. They also direct the clinician to be sensitive to child perspectives so that these are not automatically overridden by preconceived and idealised goals that come from outside the child and the communicative task at hand. One of the oldest educational dictums directs us to teach children, not our subject matter; and another tells us to individualise instruction. Attention to the psychological presuppositions inherent in child utterances helps us to operationalise these educational tenets in language programming efforts.

Speakers' Social Relationship to Receivers

The data in pragmatics tell us that even young children are at least minimally aware of the fact that communicative utterances are influenced by a speaker's perception of his or her relative social status to that of a listener. Andersen (1977) notes that four-year-old American boys, when asked to talk like a 'doctor', seem, automatically, to lower their voices and ' . . . adopt a Viennese accent'. Andersen's data also indicate that young children can discriminate between 'mommy-talk' and 'daddy-talk'. We see more and more evidence of the effects that social roles have on language utterances as we begin to better understand sexism in our various languages. With these sensitivities, we can better understand why older mentally retarded children, who have mastered acceptable syntactic forms, might still be clearly treated as deviant communicators when they fail to use polite forms and other appropriate register markers when talking to adults.

The factors reflected in these examples are subsumed in a special class of variables that Bates (1976) labels 'pragmatic presuppositions', that is, those judgements about how things need to be said in order to be *appropriate* to a particular listener or in a particular social context. Normal speakers make these judgements routinely and their influence is manifest in the syntax, intonation and lexicon used in specific communicative efforts. Normal speakers have several language codes or registers that they use; their choice of these codes is heavily influenced by their judgement of appropriateness of various codes to the particular receiver involved. Again, it would seem apparent that language remediation efforts should include some specific and systematic representation of this source of differential communicative behaviours. Current remedial models include these factors at only the most incidental levels, in dramatic contrast to the natural caregiver who, as language teacher, instinctively begins to model and reward polite forms and offer remands to children when they violate the pragmatic appropriateness rules which obtain in natural environments (e.g. 'Say please.' 'We don't say "hey you" to grandmamma.' 'We don't use those kinds of words.' 'Say doggie, Mr. Jones doesn't know what you mean when you say "Arfy" instead of doggie.').

Rules for Communicative Events

Although most competent adults and children follow the basic rules of discourse, these have remained essentially unspecified and under-represented in remedial language programmes. Yet violations of discourse rules are highly obvious and can be extremely costly in terms of frustrating the attainment of successful interaction and evoking punishing consequences from listeners. McLean, Snyder-McLean, Sack and Decker (1982), in reviewing the literature on such discourse rules in Western cultures, have summarised these as follows:

(i) Speakers must be *efficient*; that is they must not give (or request) more information than is needed to negotiate successfully their referent or proposition;

(ii) Speakers must be *effective*; that is they must provide information that is adequate to specify the referent or proposition;

(iii) Speakers must be *appropriate*; that is they must use language that reflects an appropriate perception of social relationships, contextual elements and cultural expectations.

As shown in Table 3.3, these three elements of discourse interact and are influenced by several elements of the communicative event, including those discussed in previous sections dealing with psychological and pragmatic presuppositions. First, the speaker wishing to communicate effectively, efficiently and appropriately must reflect sensitivity to the immediate physical context of the utterance in that it should be relevant to the context. He or she must distinguish the intended referent from other potential referents in the immediate context and should assume information already available to the listener in the context. Second, utterances should be effective, efficient and appropriate in terms of their relationship to previous elements in the conversation. Thus utterances should come at appropriate times, adjacent to utterances of the listener. They should assume referents already identified in previous parts of the conversation by pronominalisation and ellipsis, and should be highly specific in introducing new referents into the conversation. Third, the form of good conversational utterances should reflect appropriateness in terms of politeness and assumptions of knowledge known to be shared with a particular listener. Thus one might identify a person as 'John's daughter-in-law' as opposed to 'Molly O'Dell'. The previously identified requirements for adequate marking of referents not known to a listener remain in force.

Anyone who has spent time with young children knows that they do not always reflect implicit knowledge of these discourse rules. The long soliloquies in which children convey every detail of a television programme are painful evidence of this ignorance. So are those occasions when children seem not to follow a previously established topic because they leap off into referents and events which are not immediately identifiable by an adult who may not be prepared for the child's particular internal schema regarding the topic. Children will often amaze one by reflecting rememberances of shared histories that have been essentially forgotten by adults. Research by Menig-Peterson (1975) shows that three- and four-year-old children are differential in the ways they relate certain events to those with whom they have shared these events and those with whom these events were not shared. Children also have high expectations of adults to remember specific referents that may have come to serve as prototypic examples of those referents by children (e.g. 'You know daddy, an arfy like the one we used to have. You mean a doggie? Yes, a doggie like Arfy.').

Table 3.3: Conversational Skills and Presuppositions

Influencing Factors	Conversational Rule: Be Appropriate	Conversational Rule: Be Effective (enough information)	Conversational Rule: Be Efficient (but not too much)
Immediate physical context	Responses reflect contextual contingency/relevance	Responses distinguish referent from alternatives	Responses presuppose information obvious in physical context
Linguistic context/preceding utterances	Responses fill turn with relevant (contingent utterance)	Responses distinguish referent from alternatives introduced in previous utterances Specify referents not introduced in previous utterances	Responses presuppose information established in previous utterances (pronominalisation; ellipsis)
History of experience shared by speaker and listener	Responses reflect appropriate language register and use polite forms	Responses distinguish referent from alternatives known to be shared with a particular listener Responses specify referent known to be unfamiliar/unknown to a particular listener	Responses presuppose information known to be shared with a particular listener

Source: McLean *et al.*, 1982, reprinted by permission.

Nonverbal Representation of Discourse Rules. Like other aspects of language usage, certain elements of discourse skills would seem to reflect precursors in early, non-language behavioural patterns. Bruner (1975) stresses the context of mother-child interaction as a vehicle for the acquisition of many of the elements which are basic to communicative routines and, later, linguistic discourse. Early, nonverbal routines, for example, reflect several elements that can be seen as preparing young children for some of the rules of discourse. Mother-child interactions are characterised by joint attention to a common referent event or object. Such routines are also characterised by adjacent turns which tend to maintain joint actions and joint attention to the 'topic' of their interactions. The responses of both children and mothers also tend to be complementary in that they reflect an awareness of the previous action of one of the members of the dyad (Bruner, 1975).

Further, these interactive dyads often reflect even the sincerity and politeness demands of standard discourse in Western cultures. We have observed that young children will often demonstrate that they have given a task 'good effort' before requesting adult aid in carrying out the task. Similarly, while polite adult discourse is often characterised by indirect directives as opposed to direct directives (e.g. 'Do you have the time?' as opposed to 'Tell me the time.'), we have observed many young, communicately competent children to seek proximity to an adult, nonverbally demonstrate effort in opening a bottle, and by uttering 'can't' or 'hard' indirectly request adult help on the task. Of course, at other times, children might not reflect such polite behaviours and adults frequently state the rules quite explicity; for example 'Wait your turn.' 'Mummy's talking, wait until she's finished before you ask her to help you.'

It has been our observation (McLean *et al.*, 1982) that these patterns which characterise the prelinguistic 'dyadic interaction' episodes between children and caregivers seem to foreshadow the elements that are later manifested specifically in the discourse rules of our culture. Thus, again, later linguistic responses and patterns would seem to map on to already established prelinguistic patterns of turn-taking, turn-filling and indirect-directive forms. This observation reflects Bruner's (1975) position that early mother-child interaction patterns serve as a pervasive and powerful context for modelling and reinforcing the patterns of human communicative exchange in order that they might be acquired by young children.

Implications for Treatment

There would seem to be little difficulty in perceiving that applications of these perspectives on pragmatics do, indeed, have important implications for remedial language programmes. Often, however, the operationalisation of these implications is difficult to attain. There is considerable interference to these newer perspectives emanating from past procedures and from past service delivery systems. For example, behaviourally-oriented programmes which feature massed trials of imitative stimulus conditions aimed at the specific topography of linguistic responses militate against the designing of interactive contexts in which specific and desired responses might only be evoked a few times. Past concentration on idealised linguistic structures militate against the evocation of responses which feature many deletions of a full response because of information that might be presupposed in a dialogue. Previous programmes which operationalised a 'remedial-logic' approach (Guess *et al.*, 1977) by targeting spoken linguistic forms with severely language deficient mentally retarded clients militate against seeking prelinguistic responses as appropriate precursors of later linguistic targets. Finally, past models which emphasise one-on-one, massed-trial procedures militate against more interactive approaches which utilise social contexts *in situ*.

Although we can be sensitive to the demanding changes that might be required to implement better representation of pragmatic perspectives in remedial programmes, we must also be sensitive to the many potential gains that might be expected if we *can* operationalise these perspectives. A rather global discussion of these potential gains will be the focus of the remainder of this chapter. These gains would appear to be focused in at least four general areas.

(i) Perspectives from pragmatics would appear to provide the bases for identifying more valid, multi-dimensioned behavioural *products* for targeting in remedial language programmes.

(ii) Perspectives from pragmatics would appear to provide the bases for identifying richer multi-dimensioned *processes* that should be reflected in the procedures of remedial language programmes.

(iii) Perspectives in pragmatics would appear to provide the bases for the design of remedial programmes which target communicative *performance* which is immediately functional in non-clinical environments.

(iv) Perspectives from pragmatics would appear to provide the bases for designing remedial programmes which are much more sensitive to the roles and contributions needed from the children involved in such programmes.

Each of these areas of potential gain will be further detailed and discussed in the sections following.

Identifying Remedial Programme Products

After studying the perspectives and data emanating from the overall field of pragmatics, one is struck by the disparity which exists between the communicative behavioural products that appear to be generic to natural language teaching and those products that are the target of remedial programmes which have been designed on the basis of past, reductionistic models. This disparity seems generally reflective of the differences between a model focused on linguistic responses versus one focused on communicative responses. The details of the disparity between these two models appear to offer some important insights for clinicians and teachers.

A behavioural-linguistic model, for example, might lead one to target various response forms ranging from words, to phrases, to full syntactically-appropriate sentences. The question, then, becomes *which* words, phrases and syntactic structures? Too often the direction of the linguistic targets have been derived from criteria which were both arbitrary and superficial, for example product goals of 'nouning', 'verbing' and 'labelling'. A communicative or pragmatics model, on the other hand, would identify target responses in response to basic questions, like, 'What events and entities does a child need to "reference" to converse with his or her caregiving adults?' 'What strategies (words or phrases) might be useful in carrying out the wide range of social functions a child needs?' Answers to questions like those posed in a pragmatics model combined with recent semantic models might suggest that severely language-deficient children learn the words and phrases needed to 'refer to' (not necessarily 'name') their favourite toys, their pets, their adult caregivers, important locations in their environment, and actions which characterise the action components of oft-experienced ritualised routines carried out by the adults in their particular environment (Bloom, 1970; Bruner, 1975; Nelson, 1974). These are very different from the nouns and verbs that are taught to label the objects, pictures and colours that are ever-present in so many clinical programmes.

Going on with examples, we can see that a pragmatics approach would insist that a clinician or teacher generate language products which are specifically functional in structuring early communicative performatives, including: *Answering* (yes/no/ok); *Directing action* (help me/please/open/up); *Directing attention* (look/big/oh-oh/meow); and *Greeting* (hi/bye-bye). While the examples given above are focused on early language needs, one can see that the principles underlying their selection can easily be extended to generate higher-level utterances for meeting both the referencing and performative needs of older children. By integrating the data from semantic research (Bloom, 1970; Bowerman, 1973; Slobin, 1973) and those data from pragmatics research on children's performative classes (Halliday, 1975; Dore, 1975; Bates, 1976) today's clinician or teacher has a rationale for selection of linguistic targets which seem infinitely more valid and, importantly, intuitively more satisfying than those selected on the arbitrary bases of the past. Realise, too, that these newer bases for product identification have empirical support from investigations of child language as opposed to past targets which were generated primarily on the basis of adult perceptions of idealised language models. Clearly, by integrating perspectives from pragmatics with our knowledge in other dimensions of language, the product goals of remedial programmes can be made both more valid in terms of 'real' child language forms and more functional in terms of 'real' child language functions.

The perspectives derived from the theories and research in pragmatics direct remedial programmers to some communicative products that have rarely been included in such programmes. These are the specific response characteristics and overall patterns that are required for satisfactory *discourse*. There are many clinical populations who are severely punished because of their inability to carry out the appropriate roles in discourse. Treatment for these clients is obviously enhanced by the fact that pragmatics makes the rules for discourse more explicit and, thus, more targetable in treatment. There is much work to be done in the development of procedures needed to target such discourse skills as presuppositions of various types, to include linguistic contingency and register factors such as politeness and indirect directives. However, there are many mentally retarded, autistic and emotionally disturbed children who would benefit greatly from such treatment, directed toward the improvement of their abilities to carry out more normalised and more effective discourse even at relatively primitive language levels.

In addition to creating a better empirical base for the selection of specific referencing abilities, performative classes and discourse exemplars for language-impaired children, the data from pragmatics suggest one other major revision in the design of remedial programme product targets. This second revision is derived from the data which track the emergence and conventionalisation of *communicative* behaviours in young children. As noted previously, these data suggest that there is a basic continuity in the movement from the early, primitive communicative behaviours and repertoires to the highly conventionalised linguistic forms and discourse patterns observed in children of 24 to 36 months of age. This apparent continuity is also evident in the development of communicative functions, in that the communicative effects sought by young children in the early prelinguistic illocutionary stages are basically isomorphic with the communicative functions that are reflected in the performative categories applicable to the language of both older children and, even, adults.

The evidence of this continuity between early communicative performances and later language performances suggests that there is a strong basis for targeting nonlinguistic communicative behaviours with some severely language-deficient children. The expectation in such cases is that attainment of nonlinguistic behaviours may greatly increase a child's opportunities to experience the socio-communicative effects that can be achieved with communicative signals and, thus, enhance a child's potential for attainment of higher-level linguistic responses. The targeting of nonlinguistic behavioural products would now appear to require programming along a three-element matrix involving response types (signal form), semantic notions and communicative functions.

For example, we have assessed severely mentally retarded adolescents and found one subset of this population to demonstrate only the most primitive of communicative response topographies (e.g. holding out a glass to 'request' more juice) and to use such signals for extremely limited socially directed functions such as imperative requests for food-related consequences (McLean, Snyder-McLean and Cirrin, 1981). Before targeting linguistic responses, we are targeting the enhancement of both the signal repertoire such clients use and the functions that they will carry out with this expanded, nonlinguistic repertoire. Thus we are targeting the natural 'gesture complex' identified by Bates *et al*. (1975) and the use of these gestures to carry out functions like requesting non-food-related entities (imperative function); directing the attention of adults to various entities and events (declarative function); and responding to questions from adults (answering function).

It is our hypothesis that higher levels of language behaviours can be better attained if a basic nonlinguistic communicative repertoire with multiple performative functions is already in place. Of course, only further research will demonstrate whether this continuity between primitive repertoires and conventionalised repertoires that has been observed in normally developing children will obtain among severely mentally retarded clients. Even if linguistic repertoires are not attained with these severely handicapped clients, it is our hypothesis that the attainment of an expanded and conventionalised system of natural gestures which can be used to carry out several communicative functions would represent important gains for this population.

Other such exploitation of the continuity relationship seems both possible and productive. Recalling Slobin's (1973) observations that new forms tend to map old functions and new functions tend to be mapped by old forms, it would seem most logical to focus on the development of a robust communicative system at whatever level seems most available to children, and then to target the escalation of that system to the higher, conventional levels which are most desirable. While this view certainly goes counter to the behavioural notions, that we should target only ultimately desired responses and avoid any consideration of precursors, it would seem that such a strategy is worthy of intensive clinical investigation. We might remember that the continuum of communicative behaviours which has been made explicit in research on normally developing children had not been widely accepted at the time Guess *et al.*, (1977) took their 'remedial logic' position which recommended against the adoption of prerequisite targets.

In summarising this section, it would seem that the perspectives derived from pragmatics are highly productive in the identification and specification of behavioural products that might be sought in remedial programmes. These perspectives integrate nicely with the data in childhood semantics and other of our past notions on the needed functional effects of language. In addition, these more recent perspectives supplement our past knowledge in ways that will allow remedial programmes to target communicative responses which would seem to have considerable validity in terms of their representation of the full dynamics of human communicative systems and functions.

Identifying Remedial Processes

Although the processes for the teaching and learning of communication and language found in normal environments cannot be considered adequate for direct clinical applications aimed at severely language-deficient clients, there are elements of the normal processes which would seem to enhance clinical practices with such clients. The most prevalent clinical application of the observed normal processes lies in the general trend toward better representation of the communicative functions of language, and prelinguistic communication, in interactive social contexts structured within remedial settings. The general rationale for such contexts emphasises both the presence of more valid antecedent stimuli, and the presence of more appropriate social consequences to the intent of communicative responses, as opposed to tangible reinforcers aimed at differential reinforcement of specific topographical characteristics. The discriminative and differential functions of such communicative contexts are emphasised in MacNamara's (1972) observation that such contexts were crucial for a child's understanding of the relationship between communicative responses and their referents, and in Bruner's (1975) observation that communicative routines are first modelled and rewarded in dyadic routines that attain *joint attention* and *joint action* between caregiving adults and children. Even beyond the empirical validity and intuitive appeal of these perspectives offered by MacNamara and Bruner, however, is the increasing evidence that language forms taught in contexts which are isolated from truly communicative contexts do not appear to generalise readily to such communicative contexts. Such evidence has led behaviourists to specify additional training which allows newly learned responses to be evoked and reinforced in settings other than those used in training (Guess, Keogh and Sailor, 1978). More recently, some behaviourists are suggesting that responses be initially trained in more interactive sessions, in order to counter the low generalisation levels attained in previous training procedures (Rogers-Warren and Warren, 1980). Specifically, they are suggesting that the conditions of language use in the context of social interactions offers functional variables which are important to the overall process of acquisition, maintenance and generalisation of language repertoires (Hart, 1981; Hart and Rogers-Warren, 1978).

These efforts to better represent, in remedial contexts, the socio-communicative processes observed in normal language learning environments, require revised perspectives on the antecedents and consequences which function to motivate and reward communicative behaviours. First, there is becoming apparent some recognition that speaker needs and desires operate to structure and set the occasion for specific communicative responses and that these needs or desires have not been well considered in previous remedial models. Similarly, it is becoming apparent that reinforcement of only the topographical elements of response form (e.g. 'good talking') does not function adequately or appropriately to represent the most basic properties and uses of human communicative systems. Instead, the perspective is growing that the remedial process must emulate more and more of the natural processes by: setting up truly communicative, dyadic contexts for treatment; planning consequences which are appropriate responses to the apparent intent or function of targeted communicative responses; evoking communicative behaviours in the dyadic or discourse patterns normally observed by language users; and targeting response forms which appropriately reflect the influences of both the physical and social contexts in which training occurs. Thus specific and idealised language structural forms become less the target than do forms which reflect appropriate and effective mapping of the intent of the speaker, in light of the physical and social factors which obtain in the communicative context structured as a training setting.

Such treatment, in which natural, social reinforcing consequences occur, and in which both internal and external antecedents function to structure a specific response toward a specific communicative goal, can only occur when the training context and training procedures reflect analogues of natural communicative negotiations of both referents and desired communicative effects. Further, only such dyadic communicative contexts and procedures can set up the appropriateness of the modelling, expansion or emendation strategies which characterise normal environments.

Obviously, such contexts must be carefully structured and controlled in order to assure that the desired and targeted responses are, indeed, evoked and rewarded at high enough density levels to assure acquisition. McLean *et al.* (1982) have suggested that such *in-situ*, 'dispersed-trial' procedures be made as systematic as possible and further suggest that there may well be occasions where traditional 'massed-trial' procedures might be needed for specific response-development efforts. If massed-trial procedures are employed as supplements, however, these authors suggest that the desired responses continue to be concurrently modelled and probed in more natural communicative siuations, using dispersed-trial procedures.

Beyond these general directions, the normalised processes offer additional and specific suggestions for the design of remedial programmes. Snyder and McLean (1977) identify some specific and consistent 'facilitation strategies' that normative research indicates adults use in their communicative commerce with young children. These strategies include modifications of language addressed to children, including length reduction, complexity reduction, frequent repetition and paraphrasing. Such strategies also reflect high levels of reinforcement of the 'truth value' of child utterances (cf. Brown and Hanlon, 1970), as well as high levels of responsiveness to the apparent intent of child responses. All of these elements of the natural process would appear to deserve empirical testing as treatment strategies in remedial programmes for language-deficient children. Similarly, the child's 'acquisition strategies' (Snyder and McLean, 1977) would appear to offer some rather specific suggestions for child behaviours that are critical to the process of language acquisition and, thus, deserving of attention in remedial programmes. Normal children typically adopt joint focus in interaction with adults. They also show some tendency to listen selectively to adult utterances which reflect the facilitation strategies identified above (Huttenlocher, 1974; Nelson, 1973; Snow, 1972). The gaze behaviours of infants and young children toward their mother's face (Bruner, 1973; Stone, Smith and Murphy, 1973) seem to serve as feedback and, thus, maintain adult interaction; and the shifting of gaze by the infant appears to function to direct adult attention (and behaviours) toward new topics and referents (Collis and Schaffer, 1975). Such attending behaviours seem to be worthy of clinical attention and would seem to offer some appropriate modifications to the narrow construct of 'eye contact' that dominates so many current programmes.

Overall, it would seem indisputable that our better understanding of the socio-communicative processes which operate in normal language acquisition can provide a rich source of detailed data which will facilitate the revision of current clinical process models for work with seriously language-deficient children and youths. The full evaluation of these revisions, however, can only come after a period of rigorous clinical research which investigates the effectiveness of the various individual and collective elements available in this knowledge base.

Communicative Performance as a Remedial Goal

Professionals involved in treatment programmes for handicapped children have become more and more sensitive to a demand for *social validity* of both the treatment goals and the treatment processes in these pursuits. In the past, the logical emphasis of much remedial programming lay in the demonstration of a programme's ability to make changes or modifications in certain behavioural domains and with certain classes of clients. Today, there is an insistence that such changes be productive beyond the training environment and that they function to make the overall deviance of handicapped persons less obvious or less disruptive to the so-called 'mainstream' of our various cultures.

In order to aim for such goals in communication, remedial programmes must reflect a detailed and pervasive knowledge of the cultural rules applied in communicative performances in the 'mainstream'. These aims direct professionals in communication to identify and target elements of communicative performance far beyond the linguistic surface forms of human speech and language. Although, certainly, linguistic forms remain as critical elements of a communicative performance, there are other aspects of communicative performance which have been essentially ignored in remedial designs. As we have stated previously, basic patterns of human interaction are deeply ingrained in normal language users, and violations of these rules are not well tolerated (See Table 3.3). Nonconformity with the conventions observed by individuals within a culture to mark referents and convey information will most certainly reduce the tolerance by non-handicapped people of those persons who are deviant. Finally, the skills employed to *maintain* communicative episodes are fully expected among other people in the mainstream. Failure to respond relevantly and appropriately to the communicative initiations of others has rather devastating effects on the general acceptability of a person as a language user.

These critical social skills are identified in the pragmatics literature in analyses of conversational postulates (Grice, 1975); psychological presuppositions, which allow ellipses and deletions of linguistic forms (Bates, 1976); and pragmatic presuppositions (Andersen, 1978; Bates, 1976) which allow utterances to be appropriate in terms of the relative social relationship between speakers and listeners. Each of these elements has an influence on the specific topography of the linguistic responses selected and deemed appropriate for any given communication episode. Each of these elements controls certain extralinguistic and paralinguistic behaviours as well: elements which convey meaning just as the purely linguistic elements do.

Clearly, the behavioural topographies and temporal patterns that represent conformity to the rules of human communicative interactions need to be represented in the targets sought by remedial programmes. Failure to include such elements might mean that even a child with an adequate and effective system of linguistically well-structured responses, will fail significantly in overall communicative performance with others in his or her culture.

Child Contributions to Remedial Programming Efforts

The stringent accountability standards placed on professionals working with handicapped children has resulted in an increasing insistence on the professional's responsibility for carefully structuring the products and processes of remedial programmes. This overall accountability demand is, of course, commendable and generally appropriate. In many ways, however, such demands have caused the professional to somewhat undervalue the child's contribution to the treatment programme. Bowerman (1974) pointed out, for example, that none of our idealised linguistic models necessarily represent a child's 'psychological reality'. That is, because a professional might identify and target language goals in terms of a syntactic grammer or a semantic grammar, there is no assurance that these constructs are at all those which are applied by a child in his or her production of particular utterances. Our discussion of many dimensions or pragmatics in this chapter has strongly suggested that many of our past and current treatment efforts reflect little awareness or consideration of speakers' motivations and strategies in constructing and producing their communicative behaviours. Thus as we move from Bowerman's point in the context of grammar, we can see that it seems also to be true in the area of communication as a whole. Even further, if we connect these observations with the semantic relations data (Bloom, 1970; Bowerman, 1973) which indicate a need to teach language which maps on to a child's existing knowledge, we can see strong support for an overall need to construct language remediation designs which reflect more sensitivity to our child clients' own psychological holdings in knowledge about the world, the language system and the functions of communicative behaviours.

The general implication of all of this concern for the child's psychological reality is that remedial models based on abstract and reductionistic models in either behaviourism or linguistics often reflect an extremely poor match-up with the reality a child brings to the programme. Because of our natural reluctance to go 'inside' a child's head, we have chosen almost to ignore the possibility that our remedial efforts might be structured toward goals that our clients are both ready for and in need of. By our application of language treatment programmes which are specified by our theoretical models instead of our individual client's readiness and needs, we seem, often, to make our commitments to our models rather than our clients. While none of this is truly representative of what our *intentions* are, an objective view suggests this is what often happens. Such a view suggests the great need for us to develop and apply theoretical models which are more complete and sensitive to the individual communicative needs of language-deficient children and youths.

In addition to the frequent mis-match between our models and our clients' reality, the perspectives offered by pragmatics also seem to emphasise another insight which is important to both our theoretical models and our remedial practices. This concerns our appreciation and our overall *expectations* of our clients' contribution to the remedial process and its goals. Both pragmatics and the most recent perspectives in regard to the role that cognitive attainments play in language acquisition, offer a strong view of children as active constructors of their knowledge and their skill behaviours. Many of our current remedial efforts, which emphasise professional accountability and which are based on reductionistic theories, have seemed to require that children be relatively passive in the context of their treatment. With antecedents, responses and consequences often predetermined for a remedial session, behaviours motivated by a child's own psychological state and needs are often labelled as 'disruptive' and professionals often punish these spontaneous behaviours in order to assure that the predetermined programme is carried out. Thus children are often relegated to roles as responders to arbitrary tasks and controlling stimuli, rather than being helped to carry out their own communicative intents.

While such criticisms may be somewhat overgeneralised here, they are expressed in order to emphasise a need for remedial specialists and model-builders to better consider a would-be communicator's needs and to remember the ultimate goal of any remedial work in communication. While, certainly, such work must aim for appropriate representations of the structure of a culture's linguistic system, it must also take note of the fact that the only reason for targeting such behaviours is to allow a child effective ways to influence the behaviours of others. When our methods and goals do not reflect this basic sensitivity, they often do not target language, but rather target only behavioural topographies which sound like language but which are not imbued with the most basic and critical hallmarks of language function. Normal child communicators do not talk (or sign) just to create syntax or to attain tangible reinforcers; they talk to have an effect on the behaviours of other people. They must be given the right and the ability to do this, and they can only acquire these through remedial efforts which model both.

References

Andersen, E.S. (1977) Learning to Speak with Style: A Study of the Sociolin-
guistic Skills of Children, unpublished doctoral dissertation, Stanford
University

Bar-Adon, A. and Leopold, W.F. (1971) *Child Language: A Book of Readings*,
Prentice-Hall, Englewood Cliffs, New Jersey

Bates, E. (1976) *Language and Context*, New York, Academic Press

―― (1979) *The Emergence of Symbols: Cognition and Communication in
Infancy*, Academic Press, New York

――Benigni, L., Bretherton, I., Camaioni, L. and Volterra, V. (1977) From
gesture to the first word: On cognitive and social prerequisites, in M. Lewis
and L. Rosenblum (eds.), *Interaction, Conversation and the Development of
Language*, John Wiley, New York

―― Camaioni, L. and Volterra, V. (1975) The acquisition of performatives prior
to speech, *Merrill-Palmer Quarterly, 21*, 205-26

Bloom, L. (1970) *Language Development: Form and Function in Emerging
Grammars*, MIT Press, Cambridge, Mass.

Bowerman, M.F. (1973) *Learning to Talk: A Cross-linguistic Comparison of Early
Syntactic Development With Special Reference to Finish*, Cambridge University Press, London

――(1974) Discussion summary: Development of concepts underlying language,
in R.L. Schiefelbusch and L.L. Lloyd (eds.), *Language Perspectives: Acquisition, Retardation and Intervention*, University Park Press, Baltimore

Brown, R. and Hanlon, C. (1970) Derivational complexity and order of acquisition in child speech, in J.R. Hayes (edn.), *Cognition and the Development of
Language*, John Wiley, New York

Bruner, J.S. (1973) Volition, skill and tools, in L.J. Stone, H.T. Smith and
L.B. Murphy (eds.), *The Competent Infant: Research and Commentary*,
Basic Books, New York

――(1975) The ontogenesis of speech acts, *Journal of Child Language, 2*, 1-19

Chomsky, N. (1957) *Syntactic Structures*, Mouton, The Hague

――(1965) *Aspects of the Theory of Syntax*, MIT Press, Cambridge, Mass.

Collis, G.M. and Schaffer, H.R. (1975) Synchronization of visual attention in
mother-infant pairs, *Journal of Child Psychology and Psychiatry, 16*, 315-20

DeLaguna, G.A. (1963) *Speech: Its Function and Development*, Indiana University Press, Bloomington, Indiana (first published 1927)

Dore, J. (1975) Holophrases, speech acts and language universals, *Journal of Child
Language 2*, 21-40

Grice, H.P. (1975) Logic and conversation, in P. Cole and J.L. Morgan (eds.),
Syntax and Semantics, Volume 3: Speech Acts, Academic Press, New York

Guess, D., Keogh W. and Sailor, W. (1978) Generalization of speech and language
behaviour: Measurement and training tactics, in R.L. Schiefelbusch (ed.),
Bases of Language Intervention, University Park Press, Baltimore

――Sailor, W. and Baer, D.M. (1977) A behavioral-remedial approach to
language training for the severely handicapped, in E. Sontag (ed.), *Educational Programming for the Severely and Profoundly Handicapped*, Council for
Exceptional Children, Reston, Virginia

Halliday, M. (1975) Learning how to mean, in E. Lenneberg and E. Lenneberg
(eds.), *Foundations of Language Development: A Multi-disciplinary Approach,
Volume 1*, Academic Press, New York

Hart, B. (1981) Pragmatics: How language is used, *Analysis and Intervention in
Developmental Disabilities, 1*, 299-313

――and Rogers-Warren, A. (1978) The milieu approach to teaching language, in R. Schiefelbusch (ed.), *Language Intervention Strategies*, University Park Press, Baltimore

Huttenlocher, J. (1974) The origins of language comprehension in R. Solso (ed.), *Theories in Cognitive Psychology*, Halsted Press, New York

MacNamara, J. (1972) Cognitive basis of language learning in infants, *Psychological Review, 79*, 1-13

McLean, J.E. and Snyder-McLean, L.K. (1978) *A Transactional Approach to Early Language Training: Derivation of a Model System*, Charles Merrill, Columbus, Ohio

——Snyder-McLean, L. and Cirrin, F. (1981) Communication performatives and representational behaviors in severely mentally retarded adolescents, Presentation at the Annual Meeting of the American Speech-Language-Hearing Association, Los Angeles, November. (Available Parsons Research Center, Parsons, Kansas)

——Snyder-McLean, L.K., Sack, S. and Decker, D. (1982) *A Transactional Approach to Early Language Training: A Mediated Program for Inservice Professionals*, Charles Merrill, Columbus, Ohio

Mahoney, G. (1975) An ethological approach to delayed language acquisition, *American Journal of Mental Deficiency, 80*, 139-48

Menig-Peterson, C.L. (1975) The modification of communicative behavior in preschool-aged children as a function of the listener's perspective, *Child Development, 46*, 1015-18

Moerk, E.L. (1977) *Pragmatic and Semantic Aspects of Early Language Development*, University Park Press, Baltimore

Morris, C. (1946) *Signs, Language and Behaviour*, Prentice-Hall, Englewood Cliffs, New Jersey

Nelson, K. (1973) Structure and strategy in learning to talk, *Monographs of the Society of Research, 38*, no. 149

——(1974) Concept, word and sentence: Interrelations in acquisition and development, *Psychological Review, 81*, 267-85

Olson, D.R. (1970) Language and thought: Aspects of a cognitive theory of semantics, *Psychological Review, 77*, 257-73

Owens, R. (1978) *Speech acts in the early language of nondelayed and retarded children: A taxonomy and distributional study*, unpublished doctoral dissertation, Ohio State University

Rogers-Warren, A. and Warren, S.F. (1980) Mands for verbalization: Facilitating the display of newly trained language in children, *Behaviour Modification, 4*, 361-82

Skinner, B.F. (1957) *Verbal Behavior*, Appleton-Century-Crofts, New York

Slobin, D.I. (1973) Cognitive prerequisites for the development of grammar in D.I. Slobin and C. Ferguson (eds.), *Studies of Child Language Development*, Holt, Rinehart and Winston, New York

Snow, C.E. (1972) Mother's speech to children learning language, *Child Development, 43*, 549-65

Snyder, L.K. and McLean, J.E. (1977) Deficient acquisition strategies: A proposed conceptual framework for analyzing severe language deficiency, *American Journal of Mental Deficiency, 81*, 338-49

Snyder-McLean, L. and McLean, J. (1978) Verbal information gathering strategies: The child's use of language to acquire language, *Journal of Speech and Hearing Disorders, 43*, 306-25

Stone, L.J., Smith, H.T. and Murphy, L.B. (1973) *The Competent Infant: Research and Commentary*, Basic Books, New York

SECTION II: SPECIFIC ISSUES

The contributors to this section discuss some of the specific issues which arise in implementing behavioural and naturalistic approaches to remediating children's language. Clezy focuses on the important topic of assessment and in particular on how communicative interaction can be objectively observed. She describes in detail the therapeutic use of interactive profiling as a means of accurately analysing verbal behaviour. The chapter includes a number of examples to help the reader implement a similar approach as appropriate. It is suggested that a wide range of language behaviours can best be analysed using this approach which will enable clinicians to plan and implement therapy more effectively.

In the following chapter McConkey gives further emphasis to the importance of naturalistic assessment for implementing language therapy. He argues that it is important to include observations of the child's representational play in assessment. This he suggests leads more directly into remediation and enables important adults in the child's life to become involved in therapy. By focusing on the child's spontaneous play, McConkey shows how it is possible to assess cognitive maturity and some guidelines are provided for the reader. In the final section of this chapter consideration is given to remediative strategies and related research is described. It is concluded that as play is a naturally occurring phenomenon, it can successfully be harnessed to further language remediation.

The potential role of parents is illustrated in the next chapter by Shelton and Johnson with specific reference to remediating disordered articulation. They consider parental involvement from two perspectives. At one level it is shown how parents can be used as assistants to help implement therapy through the use of selected techniques. At another level it is noted that it may be the parental interactions with their children that are inappropriate, and in such cases the role for the clinician is to foster more appropriate interactions. From an extensive review of the literature, they come to the optimistic conclusion that there is sufficient evidence to encourage further research and greater clinical applications of these findings.

The final chapter in this section introduces the reader to the possible uses of communication supplements. Davies describes the range of speech supplements available and those children likely to benefit from their use. There are two important considerations in the use of supplementary systems which are implicitly referred to. Firstly, there is the problem of accessing, that is operating the systems, which requires careful well planned learning programmes. The use of behavioural techniques to achieve this end would seem to offer considerable optimism. The second issue is acceptability, that is the extent to which the supplementary systems can be assimilated into the child's natural environment. Clearly, it is important to take into account the range of situations in which they will be used and the particular functions they will be expected to fulfil. It is shown by Davies that a great deal of practical research still needs to be undertaken before these two important topics can be fully understood.

4 INTERACTIVE ANALYSIS

Gillian Clezy

Subjectively I felt a long time ago, as explained in Clezy (1979), that working with mothers often 'worked' yet I did not really know why it worked or what it was that worked. The whole approach adopted was intuitive rather than researched. The mothers 'appeared' to love the involvement and the children 'appeared' to improve more quickly than in traditional therapy. The significant and dangerous word here is 'appeared' as at the time there was little researched evidence to support my intuitions. Recently, the literature covering child language, discourse and mother language has added much to this intuition and it has become apparent why some of the methods have been successful. This still continuing explosion of theoretical knowledge cannot be ignored and must be constantly applied and developed within our clinical practice. Not all the findings will apply to every child but some will work.

However, even then it is not enough to say 'we are doing it' or 'it works'. Research and discussion indicate that we need an economical method of recording and of qualifying and quantifying — a method which will be reliable, quicker than traditional sampling, naturalistic, incorporates the communicative dyad and is longitudinal in approach. The data so collected needs to be stored for comparative analysis and memorised for future application, especially if the clinical strategy employed can be objectively seen to have worked. The data needs to give us something which we can measure against the normative. We need to know not only about patients 'psychoneurological' status but also whether their current experiences are appropriate in fostering development, and if not, at which level to intervene and whether this intervention will work. There are going to be many problems with such an analysis, mostly because the ordering of certain factors in communication and their relative importance are not yet clear. There are, however, apparent 'universals' which research has indicated again and again and it is on these that this chapter dwells. These universals include the need for the common referent, deixis (pointing), the importance of the dyad, the role of motivational reinforcement in language learning, the importance of cognition before syntax and the place of prosody.

85

With the introduction of computers we also need to take a look at the future and realise that the data banks now available to us will mean that every bit of clinical practice and data can be used to contribute to a corpus of theoretical knowledge. The clinic can produce far more knowledge than it has in the past but the traditional case file and history writing need to give way or incorporate a less narrative, clumsy and time-consuming form of documentation. For our profile of information we need facts and figures for analysis.

This chapter describes a means of interactive analysis which I have developed in an attempt to fulfil some of these needs and which can become part of the overall assessment procedure.

The Assessment

The argument is therefore that the assessment should not only include case history reports and tests, although these are of course important, but also an observational system which looks at the elements of communication and listener variables. This should examine the subjects not only at one point in time but on progressive occasions. The analytical framework should allow for naturalistic phenomena, including interactions of persons with the environment and each other, and for sequential stages of development. The system should indicate a point of entry on a scale where intervention may be initiated in relation to specific tasks or communication skills. Later, the same method of observation should indicate if, when, and possibly how that behaviour was acquired and whether it and others have been appropriately maintained and generalised.

The Interactive Profile

For this kind of observation we need a means by which we can record, categorise, qualify, quantify and compare the data. Here we have a problem because there are so many factors which can be analysed even in the simplest interaction. Some are verbal, others nonverbal. There are, for example, elements of cognition, syntax, semantics, phonetics, prosodics, pragmatics, motivation and learning. All must be accounted for if we are to acquire as complete a picture as possible. Also, as has been explained before, our system must encompass both members of the dyad in a naturalistic environment.

Clezy (1979) introduced a Reinforcement Profile which was adapted from Boone and Prescott (1972). At the time the intent was to study reinforcement and learning rates in mother-child interaction. Based on the ideas of Dale (1976) that all language and speech trials need motivational reinforcement, Clezy's (1979) profile was developed to show how reinforcement could be modified and was closely linked to subsequent learning rates. The idea was that any effort made should be acknowledged and reinforced without a negative response, even if the behaviour was 'wrong' in the adult's eyes. In that text, parental anxiety was outlined as one of the main reasons for detrimental reinforcement schedules and resulting poor interactions. May (1967), Jersild (1968), Kahan (1971) and Nijhaven (1972), have all described the dangers of parental anxiety which is immediately transmitted to the child and so affects behaviour which in turn reacts negatively upon the mother. Likewise, Seligman (1975) and others have described a state of 'learned dependency', which comes about when persons learn that their actions have no effect in their environment, which induces a negative cognitive set and reduced initiative. As Bloom and Lahey (1978) point out, where there is a language-disordered child, language facilitation techniques should reinforce any attempts at communication whether verbal or nonverbal, and that 'use' is probably learned best in a warm accepting atmosphere. My clinical experiences showed that by improving the reinforcement schedules of the mother, the child's performance improved, and the detrimental, contagious anxiety was reduced. This was a simplistic approach but the learning rates scored on many profiles supported the hypothesis, and by the simple procedure of showing the mother how to acknowledge her child's efforts, and helping her to have realistic expectations, the whole interaction changed from being extremely damaging and negative to one of mutually positive interchanges.

The overall goal for all therapy based on this hypothesis was that little learning could take place without motivational reinforcement from the other member of the dyad or from the experience itself. Continued observation, therefore, took place to decide if intervention and modification were necessary at this level. We needed to make sure that the mother-child interactions were mutually satisfying prior to turning our attention to other tasks which might be speech and/or language oriented. The whole rationale was that unless the interaction was satisfactory at this level nothing else would be achieved with ease. In nearly all the instances of 'clinical' children I have observed, the need for this level of intervention has been necessary to some degree.

Despite the apparent clinical success of this Reinforcement Profile (Clezy, 1979), there were problems, and these were mainly due to the terminology used. Although the text acknowledged the needs of the child to experiment, experience and make mistakes (see Ginsberg and Opper's 1979 account of Piaget), the profile used the categories of 'teaching' and 'learning'. Somehow this seemed to suggest that the mother is the prime instigator of the interaction, whereas often the child is the initiator; in fact it subscribed altogether too much to a teaching model. By using the term 'teaching' we assume the mother does teach and yet as so beautifully described by Brown (1977), this seems to be the least of her roles within the dyad; although Tough (1977) maintains that the mother does 'teach'. Furthermore, the 'feedback' from the original text suggested that I had assumed that the mother caused the child's problems rather than that the dyad was mutually reinforcing with cause and effect working in both directions.

This was not the intent, any more than it was the intent to suggest that all speech and language problems hail from the environment and/or the mother's behaviour. It was, however, the intent to shift the diagnosis and observation from the presenting child or person to the dyad and to look at the effect of each upon the other. It might be assumed that the child's or patient's 'neurophysiology' was being ignored. This was not the case: the 'neurophysiological' aspects are dealt with copiously elsewhere, they are acknowledged and not ignored herein. However, having acknowledged this, then the behaviour of the subjects and their interactions with others and their environment must all be measured along with the traditional diagnostic material. Only then will the communication elements of that problem be properly handled. A teaching/learning dichotomy is not, however, the right framework in the light of current findings, despite Tough's (1977) suggestion. It may be slightly more appropriate to the clinician/patient but still the author now thinks it is the wrong terminology and should be changed whilst still retaining the profile. As a result a revised profile is presented entitled 'The Lincoln Interactive Profile' (see Figure 4.1).

The Populations of the Profile

Each line of the profile is allocated to a specific member of a communicative dyad. In Figure 4.1 we can see that the people provided for in the analysis are identified on the left by the letters M/T/S/ and C/ or P/ which stand for Mother, Therapist, Spouse, Child or Patient,

Figure 4.1: The Lincoln Interactive Profile

Motivational Activity	M/T/S			
Appropriate Cue/Response	C/P			
Intervention	M/T/S			
Inappropriate Cue/Response	C/P			
Negative Activity	M/T/S			
Turn Event		1	2	3

Key: M/T/S   Mother/Therapist/Spouse
      C/P   Child/Patient

respectively. Each clinician using the profile may decide on their own titles, but it is worth allowing space for a short discussion on why these specific groups of persons have been chosen here. The letters /M/T/S/C/ and /P/ differentiate groups of people rather than specific persons and the title name was decided upon to allow for different letters to depict each group.

In discussing whom to assess it is tempting to write here 'any child with a communication disorder', or one who is at risk for this; the reason being that we are increasingly turning our attention to prevention rather than cure. Those of us dealing with developmental disorders are particularly keen to adopt early intervention strategies to pre-empt any problems which we know might develop. Yet whoever we treat, at whatever age we treat, and whatever their problem, we need to find that population. To do this we may have to screen; but screening itself brings about many problems which are succinctly discussed by Scott (1978). He suggests that 20 per cent of schoolchildren may have problems which significantly interfere with normal progress; yet to screen for these children it would be almost impossible to set up procedures which would pinpoint *what* was to be measured or indeed *how* and *when* to measure it.

Furthermore, the costs of identifying populations in terms of risk registers, screening or even individual tests in 'identified subjects', is prohibitive (Clezy, 1976; Clezy, Brown and Moore, 1983). The benefit gained is doubtful, because so many identification programmes are not necessarily followed by appropriate intervention, or the numbers identified in terms of those tested are so minimal. Furthermore, those 'identified' may have identified themselves through the course of time in any case so the measure of 'time' saved remains hypothetical.

When considering all these problems one wonders, therefore, how to deal with current issues in early identification, prevention and optimum intervention. One of the ways these problems can be overcome is by looking at all those who have in some way identified themselves, or been identified as in need of assessment, for whatever reason. Such people are represented by the letter /C/ on our profile (or /P/ in the case of the adult). They may have been referred but this referral and/or case history will not indicate the type of intervention needed in terms of communication and their environment, or where that intervention should start or if that intervention is succeeding. The analysis described here is intended to help overcome this problem.

Mother (M) and Spouse (S) Groups

Ideally we could have called this group the 'Caregiver' group. The only reason this has not been adopted is that Caregiver and Child (and for that matter Clinician) all begin with /C/ and our groups would become totally confused. The person depicted in this group is the one with whom the child will communicate for the greater part of the time. This is not the clinician but is frequently the parent, grandparent, sibling, child-minder or spouse, in the case of an adult. The strategies this person uses, whether it be listener variables, communication initiators and responses or syntactic forms, are all seen as important in shaping the child's speech or language and therefore must be included in the analysis.

Above all the underlying aim is that the caregiver should become the agent for our collective expertise whenever possible, for it is with the caregiver that the communicately disordered have to live. It is the caregiver who will spend the major part of the time with that subject, not the clinician. It is the caregiver who is within the subject's naturalistic environment. It is the other member or members of the dyads whose interactions will shape the development of the subject. Our collective skills as clinicians should be aimed, where appropriate, towards assessing, intervening and measuring improvement in interactions in both members of the dyad within their natural environment. Likewise, if we can interact at an optimum level with our client, we should be analysing what it is that is bringing about our success and how it may be reproduced in the caregiver. We should be able to demonstrate that skill at a level at which unimpaired members of the dyad can understand it and then introduce it into their own interactions. We must then assess and see if our goal for improved communication has not only been achieved, but is in fact maintained and beneficial as a communicative skill. We must, however, be able to qualify and quantify our results and intervene, modify and measure the behaviours demonstrated by each member of the dyad where necessary.

Therapist (/T/)

In the days of the medical model (which we who manage the cognitively or communicatively impaired seem to find extraordinarily hard to modify or shake off) our jobs were comparatively clearly defined. Subjects invariably presented themselves to the physician with a problem and some state was diagnosed which directed any ongoing referral, educational or rehabilitative placement. If the physician saw speech and language as the prime deficit the speech therapist became involved; if there was a physical deficit the physiotherapist; a query about intellectual development the psychologist; hearing, the audiologist; and a personality disorder the psychiatrist; and so on. On some occasions a multi-disciplinary team was called upon, which can result, and still does unless carefully handled, in a plethora of opinion on diagnosis and management and utter confusion and exhaustion for the subject. There may be endless diagnostic sessions while the 'label' is chased; and a serious delay in constructive intervention. It is a rare occasion that allows for the assessments and intervention to take place in a naturalistic, normal, or at least representative, environment. However, in the light of our current knowledge, can we really maintain such clearly defined professional boundaries? Scott (1978) cites Hobbs' (1975) work in this area and discusses the problem of which professional procedures shall be carried out by whom, and suggests that this has become a very real contemporary issue which cannot be disregarded or handled in the traditional manner.

Frequently, when I have talked to students and others about intervention in the management of severe parental anxiety in the case of a profoundly communicatively disordered child, the comment has been 'but shouldn't a counsellor handle that?' Yet if counsellors 'handle that' what do they necessarily know of the focus for the anxiety, that is the communicative disorder? Furthermore, does the patient really always want to have two or more appointments, relate to two people, have to pay for or have the economy pay for two visits where a cohesive approach might realise the same end?

In talking of the Therapist (/T/), therefore, the author takes the stance so aptly described by Wilson (1978) and uses the terms 'researcher/clinician' or even 'researcher/assessor' which 'do not necessarily reflect different persons; in fact from the point of view of the developmentally disabled some of the most important advances have occurred when these roles merged into a team effort or were assumed by the same person' (Wilson, 1978, p. 38). So it is that we are not talking so much of specific disciplines but of the differing and changing roles undertaken by many of us from many allied disciplines. For the purposes of our analysis this person or their role is represented by a /T/. By using either /M/, /T/, /S/, /C/ and /P/ it is possible to allocate a line on the profile to any member of a communicative dyad.

The Six Categories of the Profile

It has been decided to keep to six categories in order to reduce the profiling task to as simple a level as possible (see Figure 4.1). Others, however, may decide to add to the categories or to change the names of the categories as they see fit for their particular purpose. Some may wish to reorganise the graphic representation in order to represent their concept of the whole more appropriately. For example, Harlan (1981) utilised the technique but reduced the profile to four categories and entitled one 'Child Care' and another 'Adult Facilitator', keeping the remaining two for 'Positive' and 'Negative' comment. This seems entirely practicable.

Intervention

The central line on the profile is so called and is a category allotted to the caregiver /M/, or clinician /T/, and is identified by M/T/S which stands for Mother/Therapist/Spouse. Intervention is defined as all those strategies which these people may use in communication. By communication we mean what Brown (1977) describes when discussing baby talk, that is to understand and to be understood: keeping two minds focused on the same topic. The writer generalises this definition to all dyads whether they are communicating verbally or nonverbally. Intervention, therefore, may include the use of models, prompts, questions, statements, expansions, repetitions: anything the person does which is neither a motivational nor a negative response to the other person's actions or performance. It may also include such critical factors as eye contact, touch, affection and deixis.

Appropriate and Inappropriate Cue Or Response

The terms 'Cue' and 'Response' are critical for the child may in fact cue the communicative interaction initially or respond to a cue from the other member of the dyad or from the environment. In parent/ child play sessions we hope that the mother will follow the child's cues rather than direct with a battery of imperatives which will in all probability depress the child's initiative and performance. There are, however, natural circumstances and controlled circumstances which will lead to a response rather than a cue and therefore in our profiling we must allow for each.

'Appropriate' and 'Inappropriate' are almost self-explanatory. If a child picks up a block and tries to eat it, that may be developmentally perfectly normal and a natural experiment, but it is 'Inappropriate' to the block's use and will have an effect on the intervention and/or reinforcer. The appropriateness or otherwise, therefore, can be seen not only in relation to the dyad but also to the environmental stimulus or semantic and cognitive content. In the case of the dyad, if the mother points to the nearest 'cow' and says, 'What's that?' and the child says 'horse', it is an 'Inappropriate' response to that cue. Even if we acknowledge that it may be cognitively or developmentally understandable the fact is that the referent was not a 'horse' and the ensuing communication will be correspondingly affected. It is probable that the mother would not allow such an 'experiment' to pass her notice; yet her response need not necessarily be selectively negative. Rather she could use an 'Intervention' which will help match the right word to the referent and thereby acknowledge the effort made.

The 'Appropriate' category is the converse. The scorer sees the communicative cue or response as appropriate to the stimulus which aroused it whether it be environmental or some cue from the partner in the dyad. Operational definitions can be specified in the key.

Motivational Activity

This category again is reserved for M/T/S people and can include the verbal comment such as 'good', 'yes! it is', 'you're nearly right this time, well done', an expansion, or a nonverbal behaviour such as a stroke, a hug, a smile, or Brown's (1977) affection component. This final component is most important and is in part the prosodic pattern which carries praise, encouragement, affection and interest.

Negative Activity

The verbal includes 'No', 'That's wrong', 'Didn't I tell you not to?' (possibly accompanied by a strong prosodic component which lacks affection). The nonverbal includes the frown, slap and impatient expression, possibly accompanied by a 'sigh', or 'tsch, tsch', etc., or an attitude of boredom and disinterest or non-attention, or just no response at all.

The Event

It is important to define the event. For statistical purposes, 'happenings' need to be counted. The event that is used in this system is simply the 'Communication Turn', whether verbal or nonverbal. On the chart this is numbered and delineated with a vertical stroke similar to a musical bar line. Figure 4.1 demonstrates this, but when actually charting it is easier not to have the turn dividers pre-entered because the length of each turn may vary considerably and a printed line will lead to spatial problems in recording.

It is important to note that a Key is mentioned, and if the data is to be reliable, it is critical that factors to be analysed are entered under the key along with the symbols to be used. Again, examples are given throughout the text, but Figure 4.2 shows a very simple chart to intro-duce the entire procedure. If one is carrying out a longitudinal analysis it is of course important to keep to the same recording for each occa-sion and each factor observed and recorded.

The Charting Procedure

Cevette (1979) and Clezy (1979) have clearly described the charting procedures. They remain unchanged. To repeat, the profile was origin-ally adopted from Boone and Prescott (1972). They were able to show that only a short sample from an entire clinical session needed to be recorded; otherwise, the balance of time would be distorted with more being spent in analysis than in intervention. They also showed that the time at the beginning and end of the session was not necess-arily representative. Boone and Prescott (1972) suggested recording 20 minutes of therapy and later analysing a 5-minute sample. This author suggests that as this routine is intended for frequent longitudinal use, and being well aware of the time pressures in every clinic, an even shorter sample be taken for each factor recorded. It is also suggested that the same strategy be used for all observations of naturalistic inter-changes. In all circumstances there is a period of settling down and then a winding-down period before the interchange ends or the activity or stimulus changes. The time selected, however, is for each individual to decide in relation to the findings, theoretical knowledge and ongoing experience. For statistical purposes, the length of time must be noted. Whilst establishing personal or inter-rater reliability, it is important either to video-record the clinical session or to have two or three 'charters' at once who have agreed on their charting procedure. Audio tapes are totally inadequate as nonverbal data cannot be recorded. The data, however, should usually be charted while the interaction takes place, particularly once the charter's skills have been checked against that of others or the recorded evidence. This will save a great deal of time and is one of the main reasons for this method being developed. It is a form of quick analysis which should halve the time taken for analysing clinical sessions when compared with traditional procedures. If this immediate recording worries the empiricist, then frequent reliability checks can be made. It is important to realise that observation can become careless unless such checks are made (Taplin and Reid, 1973), but they will be costly and time-consuming and not necessarily directly beneficial to the patient if the margin of error is small. The camera, incidentally, may be no more reliable than the charter's immediate penning of an interaction. Many of the problems of reliability, which will certainly be applicable to this coding system, are clearly outlined in Ramey, Farran and Finklestein (1978). Awareness of the problems may well help to eradicate them. Having settled on the time intended, and the factors to be charted, which *must* be entered in the Key, the charter merely observes the dyad communicating and marks each event or turn in the appropriate category as demonstrated in Figures 4.2 and 4.3. In these examples a dot is used to represent each activity.

Figure 4.2: Mother and Child with Animal Form Board (Pig and Horse)

Motivational Activity M/T/S								
Appropriate Cue/Response C/P	●							
Intervention M/T/S		Wh ●		Wh ●		Wh ●		
Inappropriate Cue/Response C/P			●		●		●	
Negative Activity M/T/S						●		●
Turn Event	1	2	3	4	5	6	7	8

Key: M/T/S   Mother/Therapist/Spouse
      C/P   Child/Patient
      Wh   Wh questions

Figure 4.2 is a very simple chart of the following exchange. The mother and two-year-old settled with a form board, the mother tipped it out and made some pleasant general comments, etc. and charting then began.

Event 1 — The child (taking cue from environmental surroundings) picked up a pig and looked up at the mother.

Event 2 — The mother said, 'What's that?'

Event 3 — The child picked up the horse.

Event 4 — The mother ignored the horse but again asked what the pig was and pointed to it.

Event 5 — The child continued to finger the horse.

Event 6 — This brought the disparaging comment, 'You don't know. Well, where does that one (the horse) go?'

Event 7 — The child tried to fit the horse into the pig's hole.

Event 8 — Sigh and frown from mother and an impatient snatch and fit of horse into the right hole.

This is not a rewarding schedule for either member of the dyad, and a few more observations such as this would suggest to the clinician that help is needed at this most important level.

Figure 4.3 shows a far more positive schedule. The chart also contains more information of a syntactic nature and could be elaborated upon. Therapists are free to use their own code for syntactic analysis; the following list, however, suggests some abbreviations for particular forms.

NOUNS — N
MODIFIERS — M (quantified by 'index' number — see Figure 4.3)
    Articles
    Adjectives
    Quantifiers
    Designators
DESIGNATOR — D
    (Full statement beginning with designator)
+ NEGATIVE — D + NEG
IMPERATIVE — IMP
    (Full statement)
VERB — V
PRESENT PROGRESSIVE — V + ING
WH QUESTION — WH
REGULAR PAST — R/P
NEGATIVE — NEG
INFINITIVES — INF

IRREGULAR PAST – IP
VERB + EXTRAS – V + E
PRONOUNS
    Subjective – S/P
    Objective – O/P
    Possessive – P/P
QUESTIONS – ?
CONJUNCTIONS – C
OTHER – O
    Passives
    Negation words
    Prepositional concepts
    Verb modifiers
    Explitives
CANNOT CLASSIFY – X

In Figure 4.3, we again have a mother and her two-year-old. This time there was also a preparatory sorting-of-the-puzzle period, with comments and explanations on both sides.

Turn 1 — The mother sat back and said to the child (with affection), 'Now, where's the dog?'

Turn 2 — The child found the dog, looked up at the mother, and grinned.

Turn 3 — The mother said, 'Yes, that's it, he's a brown dog, he's sitting. What's he doing?'

Turn 4 — The child answered, 'itting'.

Turn 5 — The mother 'up-graded' the articulation and accepted the answer as 'sitting' and said, 'Yes, he's sitting just like Freddy (presumably the family pet) does.'

Here we appear to have a far more rewarding interaction than that in Figure 4.2 for both members of the dyad.

The charting procedure is not difficult and can be kept to a very simple format. The clinician can add more as greater expertise is gained and the choice will depend on which data is seen as important given the current stage of development. It is necessary to see if the prerequisites are there for whatever stage the patient is hypothesised to have reached or be entering into. It must also be decided whether or not the conditions are there for those prerequisites to have been acquired; it is inevitably a 'which comes first . . . ' conundrum. Early

Figure 4.3: Mother and Child with Animal Form Board (Dog)

		1	2	3	4	5
Motivational Activity	M/T/S			•		Exp •
Appropriate Cue/Response	C/P		•		V+ing •	
Intervention	M/T/S	Wh •		M²N.V+ing Wh •		
Inappropriate Cue/Response	C/P					
Negative Activity	M/T/S					
Turn Event		1	2	3	4	5

Key: M/T/S = Mother/Therapist/Spouse   M = Modifier
     C/P = Child/Patient   V+ing = Present Continuous
     Wh = Wh questions   Exp. = Expansion

observation and analysis will help find the answer.

The dilemma of when, where and how to take a sample focuses on the validity of the clinical versus the home sample, naturalistic versus goal-oriented interactions, and the differences of having the assessor seen or unseen. There are many differences due to differing subject matter, opportunity and interactive styles. The easy way out is to suggest that the more profiling we do in a number of different situations, the more data we shall have on which to base our future practices. Lund and Duchan (1983) describe many interesting ways in which children's language may be elicited naturally. Some of their suggestions as to how the activity might elicit the sample will apply equally to the dyad and this profiling technique. At present it seems sensible to suggest that the clinician should observe in a place which is as natural as possible for all concerned, but which is time, cost and energy effective. The results may then be compared or contrasted with other situations and variables which might have a profound effect on the interactions. For example, the presence of a dominating and anxious grandmother or a favoured sibling may have an effect, and analysis with that variable both present and absent, needs to be taken to find out if the hypothesised effect is a reality.

The place and people are not the only variables which will produce differing results. Snow, Aulman-Rupp, Hassing, Jobse, Joosten and Forster (1976) and Snow (1972) found that mother's speech varied considerably in differing situations such as free play versus book-reading. Snow (1977) also cites Bakker-Rennes and Hoefnagel-Höhle (1974), who compared caretaking situations such as dressing with free play and found that mother's speech was more complex in free situations and most complex in 'book-reading' interchanges. The speech that a mother uses is defined by the situation in which the dyad finds itself. The clinician observing should be aware of this, and by ratifying it through controlled observational analysis, has the opportunity to provide far more information than we have already about such variables.

Many people have commented, particularly during workshops and practical sessions organised by myself, that by analysing both members of a dyad, one is creating a very threatening situation for the 'unimpaired' member, that is the mother or the spouse. To the writer such comments suggest just how far we have become 'brainwashed' by the medical model and demonstrates how little we understand communication. If we really are to help we must shift this emphasis. The skill of the clinician is the all-important factor here. It can be threatening for a child or adult with neurological deficits to undergo a battery of tests. It depends on our skill to make it otherwise. So it is with our observation tactics with both members of the dyad.

Specific Factors which can be Profiled

One chapter does not allow for detailed graphs of all the possible interchanges, but brief suggestions can be made for the charting of different variables which are extremely pertinent to communication. Some examples are listed below, although more detail is given for the first as a guideline for the clinician. There will be many factors that clinicians need to analyse. All that is then needed is a symbol to represent the behaviour on the chart and a knowledge of the associated developmental norms for comparison with the data required. If no norms are available, data collection is all the more valuable, as that very data may eventually provide clinicians with further theoretical and statistical knowledge.

Cognition, Semantics and the Common Referential Cue

When looking at cognition, we cannot possibly identify a single communicative strategy to observe and remediate. There are many and this again leads to organisational problems. The ensuing listing and emphasis is therefore random. There are also many factors or elements which other clinicians are aware of which are not included here. However, whatever factor it is in a communicative context the clinician should be able to score, observe, record and remediate in a somewhat similar fashion.

We are looking primarily at the dyad. If, therefore, we have a pre-linguistic infant and caregiver referred for our attention, cognitive processes are going to be all important, and communicative processes will be closely interrelated. How can we look at these? As Brown (1977) has indicated, in 'baby talk', two minds when communicating must be focused on the same topic. This in turn will develop the semantic element of the language which results. The semantic symbol cannot develop meaningfully without the referent. There are no absolute rules or definitions for the 'same topic' or for the concrete here-and-now versus the abstract, but there are guidelines which can be followed in our observation and charting.

Bruner (1976) has emphasised this need for the common referent and described in his study how the mother and child build up their communication around their joint attention and reference. Muma (1981) also emphasises that the clinician must find out what happens in establishing the joint referent. Bloom and Lahey (1978) emphasise the same point in their 'content/form' description, and here we discussing the 'content'. To quote from their text (p. 573), 'The facilitator's task is to provide experiences that clearly demonstrate certain concepts while providing the linguistic forms that code these concepts at a time when the child is attending to both'. Joint action is important, particularly when it covers syntax. It is obvious to us then that this is critical and we must see if in fact our dyads are doing what the researchers suggest is critical to language development. Not all mothers are good at establishing joint action or common referent interactions.

We may examine a hypothetical mother and infant who are together in the family kitchen. Mother is preparing the vegetables and infant is in a bouncer chair on the table at her side. The clinician watches and scores, noting if the mother talks about something the infant is tuned into or not. The clinician can even define a specific modality breakdown, that is, whether the mother is allowing the infant visual, auditory, and/or tactile stimulation. In Figure 4.4, a simple format of the hypothetical interaction is shown.

Event 1 — The infant is pulling at a thread on his jumpsuit. (He has seen it, therefore the clinician sees this as appropriate to the stimulus.)

Event 2 — Mother says, 'Oh, these carrots are tough!'

Event 3 — The infant glances at the mother, but not at the carrots, and then back at the thread and pulls a big piece out.

Event 4 — The mother sees this and says, 'Don't do that, that's naughty!', and frowns and taps the infant's hand, but she *is* talking about the common referent.

Event 5 — The infant cries at mother's 'scold'.

Figure 4.4: The Common Referent (Thread and Carrots)

Motivational Activity	M/T/S					
Appropriate Cue/Response	C/P	●		− ●		+ ●
Intervention	M/T/S		− ●			
Inappropriate Cue/Response	C/P					
Negative Activity	M/T/S				+ ●	
Turn Event		1	2	3	4	5

Key: M/T/S   Mother/Therapist/Spouse
      C/P   Child/Patient
      +   Comment or focus on common referent
      −   Comment or focus on different referent

Figure 4.5 illustrates a different chart resulting from the same environmental situation.

Event 1 — This time mother still peeling the carrot says, 'What have I got?', holding one up.

Event 2 — The baby looks at the carrot and puts its hand out, glancing up at mother.

Event 3 — Mother passes the carrot over.

Event 4 — Baby looks at it then challengingly puts the carrot in its mouth.

Event 5 — Mother says, 'Does that taste good?'

Event 6 — Baby chews on.

Event 7 — Mother says, 'That's good, they're good for you. I'll get another for me.'

Event 8 — Baby's eyes follow mother getting another from bag.

If the baby had thrown the carrot on the floor rather than chew it the clinician might have termed Event 4 as an 'inappropriate cue or response' and certainly the resulting reinforcer would have been interesting!

Figure 4.5: The Common Referent (Infant Eats Carrot)

		1	2	3	4	5	6	7	8
Motivational Activity	M/T/S							+●	
Appropriate Cue/Response	C/P		+●		+●		+●		+●
Intervention	M/T/S	+●		+●		+●		+●	
Inappropriate Cue/Response	C/P								
Negative Activity	M/T/S								
Turn Event		1	2	3	4	5	6	7	8

Key:　M/T/S　Mother/Therapist/Spouse
　　　C/P　　Child/Patient
　　　+　　　Comment or focus on common referent
　　　−　　　Comment or focus on different referent

The above profiles need not be seen as a necessary basis for immediate intervention, although bearing in mind the prerequisites of establishing a common referent and motivational reinforcement (Dale, 1976), one would assume that the kind of interaction shown in Figure 4.4 would not be beneficial at a prelinguistic stage in communication. A side benefit of this type of profiling is that when scoring the results of a timed sample we should be able to come up with a figure which gives us some sort of concept of the 'Cognitive Tempo' — a term used by Muma (1981). This indicates the rate and accuracy of information processing, but along with this, we are able to see some of the factors which influenced that 'Tempo'. Clezy (1979) termed this aspect 'learning rates'.

Having observed repeated interchanges along the lines indicated in Figure 4.4, the therapist might show the mother how she can modify her side of the dyad's strategies to improve the 'whole'. It is a very simple procedure for the clinician to show a caregiver how to follow what a child is doing with what is being said. In modifying the interaction outlined in Figure 4.4 one might follow the child's cue and change the interaction to the following.

Event 1　−　The infant pulls the thread.
Event 2　−　Gently the mother follows the infant's action and says, putting her hand there, 'What have you got there?'
Event 3　−　Both inspect the thread. (Note simultaneous turn.)
Event 4　−　The mother reverses the thread through the cloth (or cuts it off) while baby looks on, and says 'There, it's gone!'

Event 5 — The infant inspects the place where the thread has 'gone' and laughs.

Event 6 — The mother reinforces, 'Yes, it's gone hasn't it? Now we'll do the carrots.'

Event 7 — The infant looks at the carrots and puts out a hand, etc.

Figure 4.6: The Common Referent (Infant Pulls Thread)

Motivational Activity	M/T/S						+●	
Appropriate Cue/Response	C/P	●		+●		+●		+●
Intervention	M/T/S		+●	+●	+●		●	
Inappropriate Cue/Response	C/P							
Negative Activity	M/T/S							
Turn Event		1	2	3	4	5	6	7

Key: M/T/S   Mother/Therapist/Spouse
      C/P   Child/Patient
      +   Joint Referent
      —   Different Referent

This profile is charted in Figure 4.6, and when compared with Figure 4.4, achieves a more satisfying profile of covering the top three lines and includes a majority (in fact a maximum) number of plusses (+) which indicate a common referent.

It is the writer's clinical experience that it is the directive caregiver, the anxious 'don't touch' caregiver, or the caregiver who is unable to pick up and follow the child's cues, who is putting development most at risk.

Modalities

Common sense tells us that no modality and therefore no cognitive process should be ignored for too long. A deficit of some sort would inevitably develop. The extremes are obvious to us in the children who suffer from profound peripheral modality impairments such as blindness or deafness, but behavioural or environmental anomalies can also cause developmental differences and deprivation. The clinician needs to see that 'balance' is maintained through the interactive processes of the dyad. The observations we make and chart may indicate to us that we, as clinicians, must intervene to achieve that balance. The decision we make as a result of our observations will have to be subjective because as yet we do not know enough about the individual differences of the use of the different modalities, or how they function intermodally through the stages of development. There are suggestions from the work of Spelke (1976) and Pick (1978) that intermodal integration develops along with cognition and the two are closely related. In any case we do know that no modalities, particularly the semi-impaired, should be ignored. If this happened it is not difficult to envisage just how much higher cortical functions would be reorganised or affected. The silent or inappropriate caregiver, the limited and restricted environment, the confined or damaged child (adult) will have an effect on the communication of both members of the dyad. To observe the differing modalities we can use our basic charting procedure much as we have done in Figures 4.4 and 4.5, but we need to allot different symbols to the different modalities used.

Pragmatics

By pragmatics we mean the function or use of a communicative act, whether it be a speech act or nonverbal strategy. There have been many proposals for lists of functions. Studies can be broad and incorporate only two or three categories, whilst some use classes of as many as 20 or more different functions. Perhaps the clearest framework proposed is that of Halliday (1975), at least as far as child language goes. There are as yet no standardised tests for pragmatic factors, yet all those interested in the area have stressed the need for functional analysis. Nelson (1978) emphasises that this analysis should not only look at a speech act as did Dore (1974), but include the interactive model or dyad. This she feels will eliminate some of the intuitive factors required in the analysis of the speech act alone. Nelson (1978) also indicates that it is important to realise that a functional analysis should take into account both the language addressed to the child and that used by the child. The Profile of Interactive Analysis under discussion allows for this.

This chapter does not propose the use of any one system exclusively, but rather that the clinicians intending to analyse the dyad's pragmatic interaction propose their own operational definitions and symbols. These should then carefully be recorded in the Key, and the interaction analysed on the profile just as before with the new symbols or focus being utilised in the place of the referential, syntactic and other codes. If a statement is to be analysed one might use /S/, a greeting /G/, an initiator /I/, or terminator (T) and so forth. All these can be superimposed on our chart as the interaction takes place.

Prosodics

The writer is only just beginning to work on this area with the profile and has hitherto found this easier to do in a structured clinical session between therapist or mother and child. This has been particularly useful at a phonetic level or articulation therapy when utilising Ling's (1976) work on babbling skills with Crystal's (1981) prosodic features super-imposed. Symbols have been developed for Crystal' (1981) categories of the Tone, Tone Unit and Tonicity, and a ± dichotomy used if such features were present or absent in a clinically-elicited model. Such charting is well suited to therapy and soon shows the clinician what is being achieved or otherwise. When working on such prosodic features they are only *scored* discretely but never *modelled* in isolation as it would be completely unnatural to do so and might produce bizarre speech as a result.

Articulation

Standard articulation therapy can be scored by using phonetic symbols on the profile. Figure 4.7 shows a profile incorporating both phonetics and prosodics. In this session the therapist is working on the articulation of /n/ as the prime factor and also the Tone Unit.

Figure 4.7: Profile of Articulation Therapy

M/T/S			●	
C/P			‒ ●	+ ●
M/T/S	/na na/ /na na/ two tone units		●	
C/P				
M/T/S				
Event	1	2	3	4

Key: Articulation   Primary element
        +   Tone unit present
       ‒   Tone unit absent

Event 1 — The clinician modelled /na/ using two bi-syllabic tone units.

Event 2 — The child repeated the /na/ four times without the two-tone units or primary contours.

Event 3 — The clinician motivationally reinforced and explained the pause in the middle and repeated the model.

Event 4 — The child repeated and was correct in both respects.

Communication Skills in Relation to Specific Aetiologies

Hitherto this chapter has described a way in which some of the findings of current psycholinguistic research can be applied and then scored, by the clinician. Specific aetiologies have not been mentioned, yet we cannot ignore all the knowledge we have acquired in the past about our disordered populations. It is interesting, therefore, to hypothesise about how certain disorders may affect specific communicative strategies which are critical to language learning. For example a cerebral palsied child's dyad may have great difficulty with the common referent due to postural limitations. The same would apply to eye contact and therefore turn-taking. If we become aware, as clinicians, of such possible breakdowns, surely we will be able to compensate for them in the correct developmental hierarchy? Vocalisation and prosodic development is probably not at risk with the apraxic child, yet how often is vocalisation extinguished once compensatory tactics are introduced? Proper use of prosodic skills matched to the common referential cue and the 'up-grading' skills of the listener might allow for far greater freedom of expression than does a communication board. The writer has 'experimented' with some apraxic children who have become silent over the years. The results have been exciting. The children firstly begin to vocalise to display their emotions, this is a release. They then match their utterances to their actions. The vowels are frequently undistorted or clear approximations, all prosodic markers are achievable and the vocalisation is then understood from the referential cue. Abstraction presents a greater difficulty, but the pleasure of such children in normal vocalisation, communication turns and rates, is undisputable. The reward to the parents, who soon learn to interpret, is inestimable. With this particular population the spontaneous utterance sometimes then produces consonants which years of direct therapy have failed to achieve!

The hearing-impaired population should not be at risk prosodically (Ling, 1976), even if profoundly deaf. Frequently, however, their correct use of prosody is completely extinguished. This suggests that formalised speech and language teaching strategies have suppressed skills which could have developed normally and naturally. What happens, furthermore, to the referential cue and turn-taking if a child is trained to watch for signs as in Total Communication? What happens also to the balance of the modalities in this circumstance, how can the visual system cope? The application of this interactive analysis and the remediation resulting, is discussed in detail by Clezy (1984) in relation to the profoundly hearing-impaired population.

With all the specific aetiologies, what happens to the reinforcement schedules of the dyad, if the members thereof look for speech and language without recognising what a great achievement lies in the acquisition of some earlier communication strategies? Probably the pragmatic application of prosodic function is one of the most critical yet overlooked in all aetiologies. Many children who are most profoundly disordered can be encouraged to use their voices to greet, demand, initiate, terminate and describe in a situationally appropriate manner; yet our race towards higher skills may, in fact, suppress these achievements. Later such children apparently have great difficulty in reintroducing prosodic skills to identify grammatic markers correctly.

Figure 4.8 presents a matrix which hypothesises which communication strategies might be most at risk for certain aetiologies. The suggestion is, that all of us who deal with such populations should begin to think of such skills and their very great importance to communication as a whole. It is believed that these should be introduced in the proper developmental hierarchy, when known, and that both members of the dyad should be considered in relation to all such skills.

Perhaps a hypothetical matrix such as that in Figure 4.8 could be made for each child; and then the hypothesis tested by scoring on the profile. The objective approach could then provide us with much more information than we already have about disordered communication skills in disordered populations. We would then have to answer one overriding question, that is was it the specific aetiology *per se* or the resulting maladaptive interactive strategies which produced the speech and language deficit? In all probability the answer will be that both contributed, but even the most profoundly retarded or cerebral palsied child can be helped to communicate with a common referent. The child can take turns, can develop meaningful eye contact, can usually vocalise, yet does not always do so, and does not always help the listener to interpret and build on the child's use of such skills.

Conclusion

Some suggestions for the profile's use have been shown but it is useful to list them.

(i) It can be used to collect data which can be compared with standardised 'norms'. For example, if a figure such as a mother is known to

Figure 4.8: Communication Skills in Relation to Specific Aetiologies — A Hypothetical Matrix for Evaluation (It is suggested that each dyad could be evaluated according to such a matrix)

Aetiology	Use of sense modalities	Turn-taking Eye contact	Common referent Deixis/gaze	Vocalisation prosody	Pragmatics	Reinforcement (realistic goals)	Language Receptive	Language Expressive	Speech Phonetic	Speech Phonology
Mental retardation	✓	✓	✓	?	?	✗	✗	✗	✗	✗
Cerebral palsy	✗	✗	✗	?	?	✗	?	?	✗	✗
Hyperactivity	✓	✓	✗	✓	✓	✗	✓	✓	✓	✓
Dyspraxia	✓	✓	✓	✓	✓	✗	✓	✓	✗	✗
Autism	✗	✗	✗	?	?	✗	✗	✗	?	?
Childhood aphasia	✗	✓	✓	?	?	✗	✗	✗	?	?
Dysfluency	✓	✗	✓	✗	✓	✗	✓	✓	✓	✓

Key
✓ Hypothetically not at risk if prerequisites provided
✗ Hypothetically at risk and potential for intervention
? Could fall into either category for innate or environmental reasons

use 'wh' questions for 43 per cent of her total content, the profile percentage can be worked out and compared with this information prior to intervention. After the clinician has demonstrated the goal in intervention, the dyad's performance can again be measured to see if improvement has taken place. Similarly if it is 'known' that a mother uses eye contact when questioning and expecting a response, this can be charted and the therapist can see if this mother does in fact do so and 'score' the record both before and after intervention. Whilst looking at such details the achievement/failure score or appropriate/inappropriate score can be consistently recorded and the charting can be used for recording comparative success and failure and maintenance of goaled therapeutic strategies.

(ii) The data collected can be used for comparative analyses between groups sharing a particular characteristic such as a specific disorder, social class, sex or stage of development such as those identified by Crystal, Fletcher and Garman (1976) or Lee (1974). The data analysed might also be used for some of the purposes so clearly outlined in Lewis and Lee-Painter (1974), such as probability estimates or analysis of variance; this latter could particularly apply in differences between dyads and groups.

(iii) The charting can be used to train observers such as student clinicians to be organised in their observation and for assessing and improving their performance.

(iv) The data can be recorded very quickly and more comprehensively than records which are traditionally kept in long narrative format. The graphic format is easy to read and the shape speedily identifies the trend of a clinical session or general interaction, that is the top three or four lines are promising. The type of data which can be collected in this manner is only limited by the skill of the charter and this can be catered for with sequential charting and training.

(v) The scored analysis could easily be fed into a desk computer to supply ongoing clinical data for either research or future intervention strategies.

In conclusion, we have now seen that much can be superimposed upon the basic profile which should help us in our interactive analysis of the communicative dyad. We have also discussed how such variables may be affected by particular aetiologies. The method used is simple and time-effective, whilst allowing the therapist to keep careful records of what is being achieved and which factors are present in the communication being analysed. There are many other factors which could also be charted. As this is not a standardised procedure it is open to every clinician to use such an analytical procedure in an appropriate manner. One can do this by inventing one's own symbols to superimpose on the profile. Hopefully, by so doing, a clinician can keep a careful record of the achievements, both verbal and nonverbal, of both child and caregiver, and so shape the interaction into the one needed for optimum speech and language development.

Our knowledge of child language is ever-growing, and to be efficient one must know what to analyse, and therefore it is critical to keep conversant with current theory and research findings. Other contributors to this text suggest many behavioural and naturalistic approaches which need to be observed, charted, scored and analysed by all of us as clinicians. We need to use an objective method in order to utilise the information we have gained for the greater benefit of our patients.

Acknowledgement

This chapter has introduced 'The Lincoln Interactive Profile'. The use of 'Lincoln' gives credit to all the students of the School of Communication Disorders at the Lincoln Institute of Health Sciences in Melbourne, Australia, who have worked on and contributed so willingly to the development of this profile. It also acknowledges the support given by the Institute to the author of this chapter.

References

Bakker-Rennes, H. and Hoefnagel-Höhle, M. (1974) Situatie verschillen in taalgebruik', Master's Thesis, University of Amsterdam
Bloom, L. and Lahey, M. (1978) *Language Development and Language Disorders*, Wiley, New York
Boone, D.R. and Prescott, T.E. (1972) Content and sequence analysis of speech and hearing therapy, *Asha, 14*, 58-62
Brown, R. (1977) Introduction, in C.E. Snow and C.A. Ferguson (eds.), *Talking to Children*, Cambridge University Press, Cambridge
Bruner, J. (1976) Learning how to do things with words, in J. Bruner and A. Garton (eds.), *Human Growth and Development*, Oxford University Press, Oxford
Cevette, M. (1979) Analysis of mother-child interchange, in G.M. Clezy, *Modification of the Mother-Child Interchange*, University Park Press, Baltimore
Clezy, G.M. (1976) A screening programme to detect 'at risk' factors for language acquisition in an Australian population, *Australian Journal of Human Communication Disorders, 4*, 146-54
——(1979) *Modification of the Mother-Child Interchange*, University Park Press, Baltimore

————(1984) The School of Communication Disorders, Lincoln Institute of
Health Sciences, in D. Ling (ed.), *Early Auditory Intervention Programs for
Hearing Impaired Children*, College Hill Press, San Diego
————Brown, I. and Moore, D. (1983) A longitudinal linguistic study of children
with a fluctuating conductive hearing loss, who may be at risk for language
and learning, Proceedings XIX Congress IALP, Edinburgh, August
Crystal, D. (1981) *Clinical Linguistics*, Springer-Verlag, New York
————Fletcher, P. and Garman, M. (1976) *The Grammatical Analysis of Language
Disability*, Arnold, London
Dale, P.S. (1976) *Language Development Structure and Function* (2nd ed.), Holt,
Rinehart and Winston, New York
Dore, J. (1974) A pragmatic description of early language development, *Journal
of Psycholinguistic Research, 3*, 343-50
Ginsberg, H. and Opper, S. (1979) *Piaget's Theory of Intellectual Development*
(2nd ed.), Prentice-Hall, Englewood Cliffs, New Jersey
Halliday, M. (1975) *Learning How to Mean*, Arnold, London
Harlan, N. (1981) Poster Presented ASHA Convention, Los Angeles, November
Hobbs, N. (1975) *Issues in the Classification of Children, Volumes 1 and 2*,
Jossey-Bass Publishers, San Francisco
Jersild, A.T. (1968) *Child Psychology* (6th ed.), Prentice-Hall, Englewood Cliffs,
New Jersey
Kahan, V.L. (1971) *Mental Illness in Childhood*, Tavistock, London
Lee, L. (1974) *Developmental Sentence Analysis*, North Western University Press,
Evanston
Lewis, M. and Lee-Painter, S. (1974) An interactive approach to the mother/child
dyad, in M. Lewis and L.A. Robinson (eds.), *The Effect of the Infant on Its
Caregiver*, Wiley, New York
Ling, D. (1976) *Speech and the Hearing Impaired Child*, Alexander Graham Bell
Association for the Deaf, Washington, DC
Lund, N.J. and Duchan, J.F. (1983) *Assessing Children's Language in Naturalistic
Contexts*, Prentice-Hall, Englewood Cliffs, New Jersey
May, R. (1967) *Psychology and the Human Dilemma*, Van Nostrand, Princeton
Muma, J.R. (1981) *Language Primer for the Clinical Fields*, Key Printing Aids,
Lubback
Nelson, K. (1978) Early speech in its communicative context, in F.D. Minifie and
L.L. Lloyd (eds.), *Communicative and Cognitive Abilities*, University Park
Press, Baltimore
Nijhaven, M.K. (1972) *Anxiety in School Children*, Wiley, New Delhi
Pick, A.D. (1978) Discussion summary: Early assessment, in F.D. Minifie and
L.L. Lloyd (eds.), *Communicative and Cognitive Abilities*, University Park
Press, Baltimore
Ramey, C.T., Farran, D.C. and Finklestein, N.W. (1978) Observations of mother-
infant interactions: Implications for development, in F.D. Minifie and L.L.
Lloyd (eds.), *Communicative and Cognitive Abilities*, University Park Press,
Baltimore
Scott, K.G. (1978) The rationale and methodological considerations underlying
early cognitive and behavioral assessment, in F.D. Minifie and L.L. Lloyd
(eds.), *Communicative and Cognitive Abilities*, University Park Press, Balti-
more
Seligman, M.E.P. (1975) *Helplessness. On Depression Development and Death*,
Freeman, San Francisco
Snow, C.E. (1972) Mothers' speech to children learning language, *Child Development, 43*, 549-65
————(1977) Mothers' speech research: From input to interaction, in C. Snow and

C. Ferguson (eds.), *Talking to Children*, Cambridge University Press, Cambridge

———Aulman-Rupp, A., Hassing, Y., Jobse, J., Joosten, J. and Forster, J. (1976) Mother's speech in three social classes, *Journal of Psycholinguistic Research*, *5*, 1-20

Spelke, E. (1976) Infant's intermodal perception of events, *Cognitive Psychology*, *8*, 553-60

Taplin, P.S. and Reid, J.B. (1973) Effects of the instructional set and experimenter influence on observer reliability, *Child Development, 44*, 547-54

Tough, J. (1977) *The Development of Meaning*, Allen and Unwin, London

Wilson, R.S. (1978) Sensori-motor and cognitive development, in F.D. Minifie and L.L. Lloyd (eds.), *Communicative and Cognitive Abilities*, University Park Press, Baltimore

5 THE ASSESSMENT OF REPRESENTATIONAL PLAY: A SPRINGBOARD FOR LANGUAGE REMEDIATION

Roy McConkey

'He's three and isn't talking.' Familiar words aren't they? You will have read them on many a referral note or heard them spoken by concerned parents, playgroup leaders or colleagues. They want your help. And so begins the process of language remediation. First, you will want to obtain more information about the child. Case-notes and interviews should yield some useful leads but invariably you will want to assess the child for yourself. What will you do then? The options are many. Your professional training and past experience will predispose you to certain procedures while time constraints will rule out others.

However, in this chapter I want to persuade you to include in your assessments, observations of the child's representational play with objects when they are in the company of a familiar adult. My arguments in summary are as follows.

(i) It provides you with an easily obtained indication of the child's cognitive maturity.
(ii) It leads directly into remediation as it lets you see the quality and quantity of the child's nonverbal representations.
(iii) It enables the child's parents and/or familiar adults such as playgroup leaders, to be actively involved in remediation from the outset.

But I realise that it is not enough to convince you intellectually, I also need to show that this is a feasible procedure to use. Hence part of the chapter is devoted to explaining how to carry out this type of assessment. I shall end on a more speculative note by examining links between nonverbal representational abilities and language competence and the implications these have for the style and content of our intervention programmes.

Three Arguments for Assessing Representational Play

Cognitive Maturity

Delays in language acquisition have to be set against the child's maturity in other domains — gross motor, social, emotional, but especially cognitive, development. Such data will help to decide whether you are dealing with a specific or generalised lag. Yet it is notoriously difficult to assess adequately a child's cognitive maturity especially during the transition from sensorimotor to preoperational functioning (Piaget, 1962). Psychologists may turn to infant development scales such as Bayley, Griffith or Cattell but these have a preponderance of sensorimotor items and may well end up underestimating the child's competence due to ceiling effects. Conversely, tests designed to assess the intellectual abilities of preschoolers — Stanford Binet, McCarthy or Wechsler Preschool — can prove equally inadequate due to their reliance on verbally-mediated items. Hence children's poor performance is but another reflection of their delays in language acquisition. Yet such erudite issues can fade into insignificance when faced with the practical difficulty of gaining an active preschooler's compliance with the test instructions. Their failure to 'perform' may stem from an unwillingness to co-operate rather than a lack of competence.

During the last decade a solution to these practical and theoretical difficulties has evolved. Detailed research into young children's free play with objects — usually dolls and accessories — has identified a consistent developmental progression. This sequence has been observed in cross-sectional (Fenson, Kagan, Kearsley and Zelazo, 1976) as well as longitudinal studies (Rosenblatt, 1977; Nicolich, 1977), in free-play (Jeffree and McConkey, 1976a) and structured settings (Lowe, 1975), and with Down's Syndrome infants (Hill and McCune-Nicolich, 1981) and profoundly retarded children (Whittaker, 1980), as well as with ordinary infants growing up in Europe, the USA and Japan (Shimada, Kai and Sans, 1981).

The five stages making up the developmental sequence can now provide a yardstick for measuring a child's capacity for representational and symbolic acts, a critical feature in preoperational cognitive maturity.

Stage 1: Presymbolic Exploratory Play Acts. For the first nine months of life the child's actions take little account of the functional characteristics of objects. Instead the infants' actions seem to be directed towards discovering the physical properties of objects — are they hard, or soft, do they make a noise or not?

Uzgiris and Hunt (1975) have made detailed observations of infants' actions within this stage and found that they evolve from gross actions like mouthing and shaking to ones like examining, feeling/rubbing, dropping, throwing, all of which require more precise motor movements under visual guidance. Moreover, during this stage the children tend to play with one object at a time and lose interest when it falls out of reach.

Stage 2: Presymbolic Relational Play. The main feature of this stage is the child's attempts to relate two or more objects; initially by simply banging them together but later by piling them up or placing them inside one another. In this early step, the children are still focusing on the physical properties of the objects. A second type of relational play also emerges. Children begin to identify objects by their use in relation to themselves, for example drinking from a cup, using a comb on their hair, placing telephone receiver to ear or pushing a model car along. The children are 'naming' each object by an action. Moreover at this point, children begin to ascribe unique actions to different objects and the same action to similar objects, that is a child will 'drink' from various cup-like objects whereas the 'push along' action will be reserved for car-like toys. A third strand in this stage is the children's attempts to relate associated objects in play such as stirring a spoon within a cup or a dish, putting a pillow on the play-bed and replacing a lid on the teapot. These presymbolic acts usually appear between 9-12 months and prior to the infant's first words.

Stage 3: Self-pretend. The first instances of pretend occur around 12-13 months, and are observed as the child re-creates an everyday event such as feeding, not just by placing the cup or spoon to the lips (as in stage 2) but by adding lip-smacking noises, licking actions and/or smiling. In Piaget's terms the child has begun to distinguish between the 'symbol' — the pretend actions — and its referents — the actions usually associated with feeding. Note though that at this point the symbol and the referent are virtually synonomous. Unfortunately the distinction between stage 2 and 3 is more real in theory than in practice. It can be very difficult for an observer to detect whether a child is pretending or merely repeating a familiar action routine. However, as the child's capacity for representation matures, their self-pretend acts become more recognisable through elaborated gestures accompanied by appropriate sound-effects and the use of substitute or less realistic objects such as combing their hair with a stick of wood.

Stage 4: Decentred Pretence. The novel feature at this stage is the child's involvement of others in the pretence. In many instances, familiar adults are the first to be brought in: the child offers a spoon to mother, feeds her, then may giggle or smile coyly. Although apparently a simple extension of self-pretending, it is a major cognitive advance, for the child has switched roles from an 'eater' to a 'feeder'. As their representational skills mature, infants begin to apply these pretend actions with inanimate substitutes for people, for example feeding or washing dolls, stuffed toys or puppets. Later still the child may make the doll an active agent of its own action, for example the doll is made to hold the cup before it 'drinks' from it or the doll walks, jumps and does somersaults. These developments usually occur between 12 and 18 months.

Stage 5: Sequences of Pretend. Around 18 months of age, children begin to link their pretend actions into sequences, thereby establishing a theme and sustaining the pretence for longer. The earliest sequences are based around one pretend act carried out with different people — child washes own face, then the mother's then the doll's. A second type of sequence involves linking different actions around a theme, such as 'bathing' — child removes doll's dress, places doll in bath, washes it, takes it out and makes it stand while drying it.

These sequences will occur initially as bursts of pretence, interrupted by other play acts, but over time the child will link various sequences in a logical order to give a sustained re-creation of various events — feeding, bathing, going to bed.

By now the children are showing many signs of having mentally planned their actions in advance. Their actions follow a logical order: they will interrupt the play only to search for a suitable object; they will use a substitute or even imaginary object; and they may even announce the next sequence, 'Time for bed now'. By 36 months, most children will be regularly incorporating the above features into their pretend play.

Conceptualising Stages

The foregoing may appear an oversimplified account of children's play development, especially to those who have tried to observe and make sense of young children's play with objects. Children do not progress smoothly from one stage to the next. Rather you can expect to see actions from different stages with frequent changes among them. How can this be reconciled with a stage theory? Flavell's (1971) conceptualisation is helpful. As Figure 5.1 illustrates, development simultaneously occurs within a stage as well as in the accretion of new stages. For example, at point 'X' in a child's development one could expect to observe behaviours from four stages: exploratory play is almost functionally mature, relational and self-pretending are developing whereas decentred pretending is only beginning to emerge.

In the period of time up to point 'Y' the following developments will have occurred: sequence pretending is beginning to emerge; the child's capacity for self- and decentred pretending has improved; and relational play acts are nearly fully matured. However stage 1 actions have completely matured, so much so that they no longer serve a useful function. Thus these behaviours drop out of the child's repertoire, although the potential for exhibiting these behaviours still exists. (An analogy could be drawn with crawling as a precursor of walking abilities.) In terms of play, visual exploration now suffices for exploring objects, but when faced with novel material, the child — just like an adult — can resort to the old routines of manual actions, tapping, feeling, turning it round, and so forth.

This model can account for the diversity of play acts you can expect to observe; but one problem remains. The boundaries between the stages are not at all clear-cut. It can still be difficult for an observer to distinguish one stage from another — was the child pretending to feed the doll (stage 4) or merely hitting it with a spoon (stage 1)? These judgements become easier to make with practice and experience. The best pragmatic advice I can offer is *when in doubt, assume a lower stage.* Meanwhile you might ponder on this — pretence is as much in the eye of the beholder as it is in the mind of the player.

To summarise I have presented a yardstick for ascertaining a child's cognitive maturity by observing their play with common toys such as dolls, action-men, cars, pretend furniture, teasets and so forth. Remember, the focus is on the child's *spontaneous* actions, not behaviour elicited by a tester. It's a procedure that can be used in any place, with any type of toys and requires no special expertise other than knowledge of children's play development.

You can expect to find impoverished representational play with mentally handicapped children (Jeffree and McConkey, 1976a), blind children (Fraiberg and Adelson, 1973) and autistic children (Rutter, Bartak and Newman, 1971). However, there are generally no

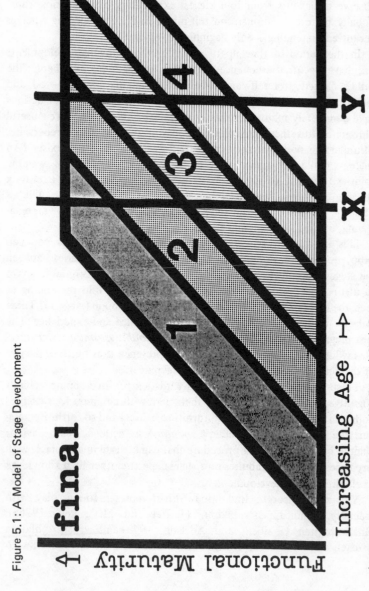

Figure 5.1: A Model of Stage Development

(Adapted with permission from J.H. Flavell (1971), 'Stage related properties of cognitive development', *Cognitive Psychology*, 2, 421-453.

delays in the play of disadvantaged children (Singer, 1973), in deaf children of normal intelligence (Gregory, 1976), of speech-delayed children (Lovell, Hoyle and Siddal, 1970), of children with cerebral palsy and no intellectual impairments (Hewett, 1970), and of children with developmental receptive aphasia (Rutter, Bartak and Newman, 1971).

From Nonverbal to Verbal Representations

'Assess then remediate' has become a platitude of our times. The truth is that few of our existing assessment procedures have been designed to lead directly into remediation (Muller, Munro and Code, 1981). For example, normative tests are designed solely to reflect an individual's standing *vis-a-vis* his or her peers. Rarely do they adequately highlight a child's specific strengths and weaknesses which could be translated into learning objectives and teaching strategies. By contrast these follow on naturally from play assessments.

The ultimate goal with all, or nearly all, language-delayed children is to get them talking meaningfully, purposefully and spontaneously. Yet this cannot happen without an adequate foundation of prerequisite skills. In particular, an understanding of objects and events (Mac-Namara, 1972), variously referred to as 'non-verbal comprehension' (Cooper, Moodley and Reynell, 1978) or 'inner language' (Rutter, 1972); secondly, skills in nonverbal communication (Bruner, 1975); and thirdly the child's capacity to comprehend verbal referents when they are used by others (Donaldson, 1978).

I want now to illustrate the potential of play-based assessments in yielding information about these three prerequisite areas and show how remedial strategies can easily evolve.

Developmental theorists such as Piaget (1962) maintain that children's knowledge about objects and events is first expressed through actions (sensorimotor understanding) and only later can they use symbols to represent reality. Moreover, all the data from developmental studies support the progression from action-based understanding to verbal expression. Hence observation of play, particularly in stages 2, 3 and 4, will help you identify the objects and events which the child recognises and re-creates. From here, you could embark upon a remedial programme which focuses on mapping verbal labels to the child's actions (Chapman, 1981). In this scenario there is no emphasis on getting the child to speak. Verbal imitation or parroting words to familiar stimuli can and does occur in the absence of nonverbal understanding. However, I suspect that this behaviour involves nonlinguistic

processes because the resulting behaviour is neither meaningful or purposeful in any communicative sense. As Rees (1975) has pointed out,
this is a trap which *language* remediators must be careful to avoid.

Language also evolves |out of nonverbal communications. Yet
remediators have a poor record when it comes to examining children's
communicative competence. Young children clam up when they are in
unfamiliar surroundings with a stranger. But the converse, observing
children in their usual surrounding with a familiar adult, is a fruitful
field for assessment. Moreover, as Dunn and Wooding (1977) amongst
others have noted, when children and adults are provided with 'pretend'
toys, the drive to communicate is heightened. 'The child involved the
mother by talking or demonstrating, or the sequence (though initiated by the child) took place when they (i.e. child and mother) were
engaged in joint attention on the same objects or material' (p. 50).
Among the communication techniques you could expect to see children
use are eye-contact, smiling, imitation, reaching out for proffered
object, offering and releasing toy, pointing, meaningful gestures such
as shake of head for 'no' and so on. Here, too, your observations will
guide the level and type of remedial strategies you employ with the
child (Newson, 1976).

Finally, joint play between adult and child will give you opportunities to observe the extent to which the child comprehends the
adult's verbalisations. For example, does the child respond appropriately
when the adult says 'now give teddy a bath' or does the child need
gestural cues or physical guidance for the message to get across? If
opportunities like these do not arise spontaneously, you can ask the
parents to suggest activities for the child (see later). Moreover, these can
be graded in difficulty from 'Give me the cup' to 'Have teddy sit in the
car and put dolly on the chair'. These observations will let you see the
child's competence at comprehension in a relatively natural setting.
Such information will be directly relevant when it comes to selecting
appropriate learning goals.

Involvement of Parents and Staff

'Start as you mean to continue' sums up my third argument for
assessing children's play in the company of familiar adults. There is a
sense in which our vision or philosophy of therapy determines the type
of assessment we embark upon with children. Therapists attracted by
behavioural approaches (e.g. Guess, Sailor and Baer, 1974) will use
different techniques to those following cognitively-based approaches
(e.g. Cooper, Moodley and Reynell, 1978).

Likewise on a wider plane, if your therapy is to be centred on every-day activities rather than within specialist settings, the case for which I have argued elsewhere (McConkey, 1981), then the assessments as well as the treatment must involve the children's parents and the staff from their schools or playgroup. We must collect at least a modicum of infor-mation on the interaction of these adults with the child. A play setting is one convenient context for doing this. It will give you a feel for their preferred style — directive, responsive, meek, forceful and you can collect more precise information, such as the frequency, length and complexity of their utterances to the child, or the type of responses they made to the child's initiations.

Armed with this information, you can give them specific advice on how best to react with the child, highlighting their strengths and suggesting remedies for their weaknesses. This can be a crucial step in effecting changes in the child (McConkey, Jeffree and Hewson, 1979). But even in those instances when it is not, I believe the parents and staff will have learnt an important lesson, namely that a child's compet-ence in language cannot be assessed adequately, still less remediated, in the absence of familiar adults.

The idea persists that language competence is a unitary ability, centred within the child, which at any point in time is relatively constant. We may even think of it as being analogous to the ability to walk or to feed oneself. But this is questionable given the widely accepted proposition that children develop competence in language through interactions with their parents (Mahoney and Seely, 1976). We should expect children's competence to vary according to the people with whom they are com-municating and the context in which communication occurs. Sadly, many of our assessment procedures fail to reflect this new thinking. We need procedures which treat linguistic competence as a varying inter-active ability (McLean and Snyder-McLean, 1978). Finally, in play-based observations, parents or other adults are not present as spec-tators. Rather they are given a *purposeful* role from the outset, that of playmate for the child, thereby leaving the therapists free to ob-serve.

Observing Children's Play

I suspect you will want to reserve judgement on the foregoing rationale until you have a better idea as to what precisely is involved in observing children's play. Hence this section gives details on how to observe play.

McCune-Nicolich and Fenson (1983), in their review of research to date, suggest the ideal assessment would be as follows.

(i) Observations are carried out in the child's home or in other familiar settings such as playgroups.

(ii) A familiar adult, preferably a parent, should be present to play with the child.

(iii) The child's own toys could be used, although these should be supplemented by specially chosen toys.

(iv) A minimum of 20 minutes play, on two different occasions, is recommended.

(v) Adult playmates should take a passive but responsive role for the first part of the session. Later they can be asked to model and/or suggest play activities which are slightly in advance of those performed spontaneously by the child.

(vi) The sessions should be video-recorded for later analysis.

If some of these conditions are unobtainable, compromises can be made, although invariably some sacrifice may ensue.

Setting

Home may be best but then it is not always practical. The alternative is to simulate home surroundings in a clinic or preschool setting through the provision of carpeting, comfortable chairs, freedom from office noises or other distractions and child-size furniture. Moreover it helps if the child and adult are given time to familiarise themselves with these surroundings. Wendy-house screens can be used to create an observation corner within a classroom.

Toys

Careful thought should be given both to the type of toys used and how they are presented. A 'core set' would include the following: two rag dolls (dressed in removable clothing), a doll's bed with 'pillow' and 'sheet'; a chair and table appropriately sized for the doll; miniature cup, spoon and comb; and a cardboard box (e.g. shoe box) which can represent a bath, car, boat, and so forth. Additions can be made depending on the level of play you want to explore. For example, sequence pretending may be elicited by providing more characters, for example stuffed animals or action-men or by adding other props such as teapots, saucepans, cookers, irons, or trucks. Equally more ambiguous material could be provided such as empty yoghurt cartons, boxes, sticks, blocks of wood. These will let you see the child's capacity for object substitution.

For children at an earlier stage, it is worth widening the range of toys that would elicit exploratory and relational play actions. For example, rattles, mirrors, nesting boxes, cubes, containers with easily-removed lids, a toy telephone and push-along cars.

The toys can be presented altogether in a box, or displayed around the room or given to the child singly or in sets. Each alternative has its advantages and disadvantages. Simultaneous presentation of a lot of toys results in a high level of exploratory actions before the child settles down to more purposeful play, whereas selective presentation constrains children to certain actions. The strategy I favour is to begin with the core set and as the session progresses bring out other toys. These can be chosen according to the child's level of play maturity.

Finally, certain children, such as those who are severely handicapped or 'autistic', may show no interest at all in toys. With them we have resorted to 'augmented' toys, that is those with bells, buzzers or lights. For example, the rag doll is fitted with two lights for eyes which the adult can flash when the child plays with it (McConkey and Jeffree, 1982). The goal of assessment is to determine what the child *can* do, albeit under the most favourable conditions.

Adult's Role

Children's pretence is facilitated by the presence of a familiar adult (Fein and Robertson, 1975), especially mothers (Dunn and Wooding, 1977; McConkey and Martin, 1983). Moreover, Sorce and Emde's (1981) research suggests that infants play more when they perceive their mothers are available, for example watching them play, rather than when they are present but reading a book or ignoring the child's advances. Hence the common scenario of leaving a child to play alone with toys in the presence of a 'detached' observer is *not* recommended.

For the first 5-7 minutes of the session, the adult's role should be that of 'reponsive spectator'. Unfortunately adults differ widely in their interpretations of these instructions: some will practically ignore the child whereas others will become so directive that you end up with no indication of the child's spontaneous play activities. Nonetheless these valuable insights into the adult's behaviour have to be balanced against information about the child's competence, so be prepared to give some adults more explicit guidance.

Models and Suggestions

Even when you have a sample of the children's spontaneous play, there remains the possibility that they could have done better. In particular, your sample is unlikely to include actions from a stage which is just beginning to emerge. Yet this is vital information for a full assessment of their competence. Experimenters have used various modelling strategies and/or verbal suggestions to elicit play actions which are one or two stages ahead of the child's spontaneous actions. For example Fenson and Ramsay (1980) modelled specific pretend sequences and then immediately gave the children the opportunity to imitate with only the necessary toys to hand. Not surprisingly, this approach elicited more pretend acts than did a variety of pretend actions modelled consecutively in a free-play setting, an approach favoured by Jeffree and McConkey (1976a). Nonetheless they demonstrated that the effects of modelling carried over into a later free play period.

Evidence for the efficacy of verbal suggestion *per se* is confined more to older children (Pederson, Rook-Green and Elder, 1981), although others have used it in conjunction with modelling (e.g. Fenson and Ramsay, 1981). This can be a natural approach to investigating children's comprehension of language as well as eliciting more advanced play. The suggestions should include actions known to be within the child's repertoire as well as ones at a more advanced level (Miller, Chapman, Branston and Reichle, 1980). If the child does not respond to suggestions alone, models can then be tried.

Thus the second part of the observation should be devoted to observing the effects of the adult's models and suggestions. However, for the final part of the session, I recommend that the adult reverts to the role of 'responsive spectator' so that you can see if any changes are maintained. If you are concerned about boredom or fatigue effects take a break after the modelling.

Recording

Video-records are best for carrying out a thorough analysis of the child's and adult's actions. It is by no means accidental that the upsurge in observational research studies coincides with the advent of portable video-systems. Nevertheless the problem of synthesising the data from video-records still remains. Fortunately the methods used for doing this can be translated into recording schedules for observers to use *in situ* as well as from video-recordings.

Figure 5.2 shows one approach. The observer places a tick against the stage whenever an action occurs. For example if the child combs

Figure 5.2: A Simple Checklist for Recording Play Actions

OBJECT PLAY CHECKLIST

CHILD'S NAME Martin   DATE 7ᵗʰ JUNE

LENGTH OF SESSION 16 Mins   OBSERVER JUDY

COMMENTS Slow to play at beginning but joined in readily when mother modelled.

STAGE	TICK FOR EACH NEW ACTION*	TOTAL	%
1. EXPLORATORY	✓✓✓✓ ✓✓✓	8	18
2. RELATIONAL	✓✓✓✓ ✓✓✓✓ ✓✓✓✓	15	34
3. SELF-PRETEND	✓✓M ✓✓✓✓ ✓	8	18
4. DECENTRED-PRETEND	M M ✓ S ✓✓✓M✓✓✓✓✓	9	20
5. SEQUENCES**			
(A) SAME ACTION	(3M) 2	2	9
(B) SAME THEME	2	2	
(C) IMAGINARY OBJECTS***			

TOTAL OVERALL

Notes: *M = Modelled   S = Suggested   Excluding 'M' & 'S'.
**Enter the number of actions making up the sequence
***Actions with imaginary objects are ticked here but not counted in the total as they will usually occur within a sequence and should be counted there.
ⓒ*St Michael's House Research*

the doll and then mouthes the comb, stages 4 and 1 are ticked, respectively. At stage 5, a count is kept of the number of actions making up a sequence and then entered as a total in the appropriate row. For example, if a boy feeds himself, then a doll, then mother, '3' is entered in the same action row. It is important to distinguish children's spontaneous actions from those modelled or suggested by an adult. The letters 'M' for modelled and 'S' for suggested can be used to do this.

The completed checklist highlights two vital facts: (i) the highest stage of play observed; and (ii) the stage at which most of the child's actions were centred. Frequency measures of this type have been the most popular with researchers yet they have one major drawback. No details are kept of the children's specific actions, which could be important information when it comes to selecting learning objectives. The alternative is to compile a more comprehensive schedule which lists, for each stage, the likely play actions children might perform. For example, the list for stage 4 might include the following: feeds with spoon, feeds with cup, puts to bed, washes, combs, sits on chair, walks, kisses. The observer then circles or ticks an action as it is observed or writes in novel actions whenever they occur. This type of checklist will highlight the child's most popular actions and also those which the child did *not* perform. Models or suggestions could be used in an attempt to elicit some of these.

These are but two examples of how detailed information can be extracted from play sessions. Needless to say different checklists would be needed if you wanted details on adults' style of interaction and the child's proficiency in nonverbal communication. Video is the only way of simultaneously recording all these facets of dyadic interchanges.

Time Involved

The play assessment will probably take around 20 minutes in total, a few minutes warm-up, 5-7 minutes free play, 5 minutes or so of adult modelling, followed (after an interval if needed) by 5-7 minutes of free play. However, I strongly recommend you to repeat these observations on a second or third occasion, separated by several days at least. This will not only increase the reliability of your sample but it should encourage the parents or staff to focus more on the child's play, thereby laying the foundation for future remedial action.

Getting It All Together

Data from your observations of children's play can be set alongside information about the child's maturity in other areas of development, e.g. the results of other assessments of linguistic competence, such as normative test scores or analysis of language usage. The next step is to plan a programme of remedial action which builds upon the child's skills and abilities towards the development of new competencies.

A 30-minute colour video, illustrating the stages in children's play and procedures for assessment, is available along with an instructional handbook from: St. Michael's House Research, Upper Kilmacud Road, Stillorgan, Co. Dublin, Eire (price £30.00).

Representational Play — a Springboard for Language Remediation

Springboard, according to my dictionary, is 'a vantage point from which to go into action'. If I have persuaded you that it is a valuable and feasible vantage point in assessment, perhaps you will bear with me as I outline its continuing use in remedial action. First, it has pragmatic value in providing you and the child with a microcosm of reality in which language can be used meaningfully, purposefully and spontaneously. Second, there is the possibility that cognitive growth can be facilitated by nurturing children's capacity for representation and, finally, the exciting prospect that language acquisition can be stimulated by developing representational play is brought closer.

Contexts for Learning Language

Remediation can only be judged successful once the children's learning generalises to everyday life. Unfortunately by this criteria many published schemes are 'not proven', even though impressive results were obtained in clinic settings. For some the explanation for the child's 'failure to generalise' is but another symptom of the child's problems, and so they have set about designing ever more elaborate schemes to programme transition of learning from clinic to natural setting (e.g. Guess *et al.*, 1974). Even a naive observer could rightly enquire why remediation should not be centred in naturally-occurring contexts from the outset. Fortunately there are promising signs that such an ethos is catching hold (Jeffree and McConkey, 1976b; McLean and Snyder-McLean, 1978; Masidlover, 1979). Yet as a proponent of such an approach, I do concede that it poses practical difficulties for therapists.

(i) The children need substantial practice at new linguistic skills yet opportunities for such do not easily arise in natural settings.
(ii) The natural environment may be insufficient to trigger new learning. Certain features might have to be accentuated such as clarifying the meaning of referents, or increasing the child's need to communicate.
(iii) The pressures on therapists to deal with more and more clients means that it is more time-economical to see children by appointment in a central location.

Representational play contexts offer an excellent compromise. Here you can re-create a microcosm of the children's natural environments, thereby overcoming the difficulties noted above. Remember, too, that various play settings can be used; doll play is just one possibility. Others, which I and my colleagues have used, are a miniature playground for play-people characters, with swings, slides, paddling pools; and a kitchen scene with people, furniture and objects cut out of felt so that the child and therapist could easily create various scenes (McConkey and Jeffree, 1982). Both these contexts re-create familiar settings, thus the language milieu surrounding them is automatically meaningful and relevant to the child, irrespective of whether it occurs within a clinic, a classroom or as we have often been forced to use, the laundry store!

There is also plenty of scope for sustained practice of new linguistic forms as repeated actions are a feature of children's play. Indeed we have devised other sorts of play contexts to give children more specific practice, for example a game of posting pictures of foodstuffs into the 'mouth' of a face painted on the back of a shoe box . . . 'boy eat sweet' . . . 'girl eat banana' . . . 'Mummy eat icecream'. Likewise children could move pictures of characters up and down a ladder, a wall or a tree to create sentences of the type 'cat up the tree'. You can, of course, choose your representational play context to accord with the child's particular interests — Subuteo footballers or cars and trains in model villages. I need hardly add that such activities are likely to be much more enjoyable for the child than picture cards or books, not least because the children are active participants rather than passive spectators. Play contexts go some small way to augmenting the conditions under which children normally learn language, for as Chapman (1981, p. 244) concluded in her review of mother-child interaction.

Input (from the mother) seems to play a demonstrable role in the 2 year old's language acquisition when it is specifically contingent on the child's initiated actions and utterances. It is the linguistically responsive environment rather than the linguistically stimulating one that should accelerate language acquisition.

Cognitive Growth

Stimulating children's representational play could well yield other spinoffs. 'There are numerous theorists and researchers . . . who believe that play experiences can, in and of themselves, cause growth in the cognitive domain' (Rubin and Pepler, 1982, p. 294). This conviction is strengthened by the results of various studies with normal children who have experienced 'pretence training'. For example, these children scored better on tests of divergent thinking such as generating uses for objects (Li, 1978); they are quicker at problem-solving (Smith and Dutton, 1979) and at conservation tasks (Columb and Cornelius, 1977). When children are involved in socio-dramatic training with peers, they become less egocentric (Fein, 1978) and perform better on problem-solving involving social co-operation (Strain and Wiegernik, 1976). Comparable research with adequate control procedures has yet to be undertaken with atypical children, but the promise of wider benefits beyond the children's play, does at least exist.

Language Acquisition and Representation

Finally, a still more exciting promise remains. Language acquisition could be facilitated through representational play. This is not a novel idea. Piaget (1962), for example, contended that symbolic play and language were manifestations of the same underlying process, the 'semiotic' function, which enables children to use 'signifiers' to represent reality. Werner and Kaplan (1963) proposed a similar common ability. Hence if this process of symbolisation could be nurtured via one mode, for example play, then benefits should also accrue in the other, that is language (Bates, 1976).

Recently, various writers have alluded to the striking parallels which exist between pretend play and language. For example, Rosenblatt (1977, p. 39) stated 'those (children) whose play matured more rapidly also learned language earlier, achieved object-permanence earlier and scored a higher developmental quotient on the Bayley Test at age two'. McCune-Nicolich (1981) in her review highlights four significant coincidences between play and language development.

(i) In presymbolic play, children recognise objects by the actions they associate with them (stage 2). Likewise analogous presymbolic vocal and gestural behaviours have been identified preceding referential words (e.g. Dore, 1975).

(ii) Considerable evidence exists for the co-occurrence of first words with children's first pretend behaviours centred on themselves (e.g. Bates, Camaioni and Volterra, 1975; Largo and Howard, 1979).

(iii) Both pretend play and language proceed from single units to combinations and the onset of two-word utterances generally follows the development of decentred pretence and the evolution of early pretend sequences (Lowe, 1975). Moreover, Hill and McCune-Nicolich (1981) found that Down's Syndrome children who failed to combine symbolic play acts also failed to produce utterances greater than one word in length.

(iv) Sequence-pretend play, which involves the planning and execution of various symbolic acts, appear to be a precursor to multiword sentences (McCune-Nicolich, 1981).

Admittedly, most of this data arises from correlational studies and is inadequate to convince a sceptical reviewer such as Fein (1981). Lots of other coincidences arise in children's development: they walk around the same time as they begin to talk and they learn to run at the two-word stage, yet no one is suggesting that these two domains are intimately related.

In order to resolve this issue longitudinal studies with a large sample of infants are needed in which concurrent measures are taken of language and play, so that the reliability of any syncronies can be established. However, studies of this type are costly and time-consuming. An attractive alternative is intervention studies in which the children's competence in one domain is nurtured, for example pretend play and changes in the other domain are monitored. As a foretaste of such research let me describe the results we obtained with 23 mentally handicapped children (Martin, McConkey and Martin, 1984).

Our aim was to encourage their use of two- or three-word sentences, especially those incorporating Agent + Action + Objects. Specially designed representational play contexts were used (see earlier) and as one group of children played, the teacher gave sentence models describing the children's actions. A matched control group of children played in the teacher's presence but with them, she used language in a generally encouraging way and gave no models of sentences. To our surprise, both groups showed significant improvements on post-training assessments and these gains were maintained on re-testing four weeks later. Moreover, various control procedures ascertained that the improvements were not artefacts of measurement. This then suggests that the play context — daily experience of representational play in the presence of an attentive adult — may have had a more potent effect on the children's language acquisition than did the teachers' models.

So how were the children benefitting? For three weeks they had sustained practice at creating relationships between familiar referents. Hence they could have become more adept at identifying and understanding relationships. For example, before children label a picture as 'boy riding a donkey', they would have to recognise the *relationship* depicted and not just focus on the individual referents. Thus before children use sentence rules generatively, they must first have a well-tuned capacity for representing relationships (McCall, Eichorn and Hogarty, 1977). Once this is established, sentence usage can quickly follow.

Similar conclusions are emerging from studies with ordinary infants. Miller *et al.* (1980) have clearly shown that children's comprehension of adults' Action + Object and Agent + Action sentences only commences around the 16-21 month period, the point in time when children's pretend play with dolls becomes more frequent. Likewise Ungerer and Sigman (1983) found significant correspondences between receptive language skills and levels of play in autistic children.

Until more data becomes available, these findings must be treated cautiously but at the very least they should make us ponder anew on the high emphasis given to speech in many programmes designed to remediate children's *language*. Rather, as Donaldson (1978, p. 38) argued so succinctly, the primary thing must be

> The grasp of meaning – the ability to 'make sense' of things, and above all to make sense of what people do, which of course includes what people say . . . It is the child's ability to interpret situations which makes it possible for him, through active processes of hypothesis-testing and inference to arrive at a knowledge of language.

Only when our assessments and remediations are attuned to the child's present understanding of their reality, can we begin effectively to help them. The paradox is, though, that the children have to help themselves. They must be active investigators and confident experimenters if they are to become knowledgeable language users. Our therapy must then nurture these characteristics by focusing on what they want to do. Even if all other arguments were to come to naught, this would remain as *the* justification for studying children's play.

References

Bates, E. (1976) *Language and Context*, Academic Press, London
——Camaioni, L. and Volterra, V. (1975) The acquisition of performatives prior to speech, *Merrill-Palmer Quarterly, 21*, 205-16
Bruner, J. (1975) The ontogenesis of speech acts, *Journal of Child Language, 2*, 1-19
Chapman, R.S. (1981) Mother-infant interaction in the second year of life: It's role in language development, in R.L. Schiefelbusch and D.D. Bricker (eds.), *Early Language: Acquisition and Intervention*, University Park Press, Baltimore
Columb, C. and Cornelius, C.B. (1977) Symbolic play and its cognitive significance. *Developmental Psychology, 13*, 246-52
Cooper, J., Moodley, M. and Reynell, J. (1978) The developmental language programme: Results from a five year study, *British Journal of Disorders of Communication, 14*, 57-69
Donaldson, M. (1978) *Children's Minds*, Fontana, London
Dore, J. (1975) Holophrases, speech acts and language universals, *Journal of Child*

Language, 2, 21-39

Dunn, J. and Wooding, C. (1977) Play in the home and its implications for learning, in B. Tizard and D. Harvey (eds.), *Biology of Play*, Heinemann, London

Fein, G.G. (1978) Play revisited, in M. Lamb (ed.), *Social and Personality Development*, Holt, Rinehart and Winston, New York

——(1981) Pretend play in childhood: An integrative review, *Child Development, 52*, 1095-118

——and Robertson, A. (1975) Cognitive and social dimensions of pretending in two year olds, unpublished manuscript, Yale University, cited in L. McCune-Nicolich and L. Fenson (1983)

Fenson, L., Kagan, J., Kearsley, R.B. and Zelazo, P.R. (1976) The developmental progression of manipulative play in the first two years, *Child Development, 47*, 232-6

——and Ramsay, D. (1980) Decentration and integration of play in the second year of life, *Child Development, 51*, 171-8

Flavell, J. (1971) Stage-related properties of cognitive development, *Cognitive Psychology, 2*, 421-53

Fraiberg, S. and Adelson, E. (1973) Self-representation in language and play. Observations of blind children, *Psychoanalytical Quarterly*, 42, 539-47

Gregory, S. (1976) *The Deaf Child and His Family*, Allen and Unwin, London

Guess, D., Sailor, W. and Baer, D. (1974) To teach language to retarded children, in R. Schiefelbusch and L. Lloyd (eds.), *Language Perspectives: Acquisition, Retardation and Intervention*, University Park Press, Baltimore

Hewett, S. (1970) *The Family and the Handicapped Child*, Allen and Unwin, London

Hill, P.M. and McCune-Nicolich, L. (1981) Pretend play and patterns of cognition in Down's Syndrome children, *Child Development, 52*, 611-17

Jeffree, D.M. and McConkey, R. (1976a) An observation scheme for recording children's imaginative doll play, *Journal of Child Psychology and Psychiatry, 17*, 189-97

——and McConkey, R. (1976b) *Let Me Speak*, Souvenir Press, London

Largo, R.H. and Howard, J.A. (1979) Developmental progression in play behaviour of children between nine and thirteen months: II Spontaneous play and language development, *Developmental Medicine and Child Neurology, 21*, 492-503

Li, A.K. (1978) Effects of play on novel responses of preschool children, *Alberta Journal of Educational Research, 24*, 31-6

Lovell, K., Hoyle, H.W. and Siddall, W.M. (1968) A study of some aspects of the play and language of young children with delayed speech, *Journal of Child Psychology and Psychiatry, 9*, 41-50

Lowe, M. (1975) Trends in the development of representational play: an observation study, *Journal of Child Psychology and Psychiatry, 16*, 33-47

McCall, R.B., Eichorn, D.H. and Hogart, P.S. (1977) Transitions in early mental development, *Monographs of the Society for Research in Child Development, 42* (Serial No. 171)

McConkey, R. (1981) Sharing knowledge of language with children and parents, *British Journal of Disorders of Communication, 16*, 3-10

·——and Jeffree, D.M. (1982) *Let's Make Toys*, Souvenir Press, London

——Jeffree, D.M. and Hewson, S. (1979) Involving parents in extending the language development of their young mentally handicapped children, *British Journal of Disorders of Communication, 14*, 203-18

——and Martin, H. (1983) The development of object and pretend play in Down's Syndrome Infants: A longitudinal study involving mothers. Paper submitted to *Trisomy 21*

McCune-Nicolich. L. (1981) Toward Symbolic Functioning: Structure of early pretend games and potential parallels with language, *Child Development, 52*, 785-97

――――and Fenson, L. (1983) Methodological issues in studying early pretend play, in T. Yawley and A.D. Pelligini (eds.), *Child's Play: Developmental and Applied*, Hillsdale, New Jersey

McLean, J. and Snyder-McLean, L. (1978) *A Transactional Approach to Early Language Training*, Charles E. Merrill, Columbus, Ohio

MacNamara, J. (1972) Cognitive basis of language learning in infants, *Psychological Review, 79*, 1-13

Mahoney, G.J. and Seely, P.B. (1976) The role of the social agent in language acquisition: Implications for language intervention, in N.R. Ellis (ed.), *International Review of Research in Mental Retardation*, Academic Press, New York

Martin, H., McConkey, R. and Martin, S. (1983) From acquisition theories to intervention strategies: An experiment with mentally handicapped children. *British Journal of Disorders of Communication, 19* (in press)

Masidlover, M. (1979) The Derbyshire Language Scheme: Remedial teaching for language delayed children, *Child: care, health and development, 5*, 9-16

Miller, J.F., Chapman, R.S., Branston, M. and Reichle, T. (1980) Language Comprehension in sensorimotor stages 5 and 6, *Journal of Speech and Hearing Research, 23*, 243-60

Müller, D., Munro, S.M. and Code, C. (1981) *Language Assessment for Remediation*, Croom Helm, London

Newson, E. (1976) Parents as a resource in diagnosis and assessment, in T.E. Oppe and F.P. Woodford (eds.), *Early Management of Handicapping Disorders*, Elsevier, Amsterdam

Nicolich, L. (1977) Beyond sensorimotor intelligence: assessment of symbolic maturity through analysis of pretend play, *Merrill-Palmer Quarterly, 23*, 89-101

Pederson, D.R., Rook-Green, A. and Elder, J.L. (1981) The role of action in the development of pretend play in young children, *Developmental Psychology, 17*, 756-9

Piaget, J. (1962) *Play, Dreams and Imitation*, Routledge and Kegan Paul, London

Rees, N.S. (1975) Imitation and language development: Issues and clinical implications, *Journal of Speech and Hearing Disorders, 40*, 339-50

Rosenblatt, D. (1977) Development trends in infant play, in B. Tizard and D. Harvey (eds.), *The Biology of Play*, Heinemann, London

Rubin, K.H. and Pepler, D.J. (1982) Children's Play: Piaget's views reconsidered, *Contemporary Educational Psychology, 7*, 289-99

Rutter, M. (1972) The effects of language delay on development, in M. Rutter and J.A.M. Martin (eds.), *The Child with delayed speech*, Heinemann, London

――――Bartak, L. and Newman, S. (1971) Autism: a central disorder of cognition and language, in M. Rutter (ed.), *Infantile Autism: Concepts, Characteristics and Treatment*, Churchill-Livingstone, Edinburgh

Shimada, S., Kai, Y. and Sans, R. (1981) Development of symbolic play in late infancy, R.E.E.C. Research Bulletin, RRB17, Gakuji University, Koganei, Tokyo

Singer J.L. (1973) *The Child's World of Make-believe: Experimental Studies of Imaginative Play*, Academic Press, New York

Smith, P.K. and Dutton, S. (1979) Play and training in direct and innovative problem-solving, *Child Development, 50*, 830-6

Sorce, J. and Emde, R.N. (1981) Mother's presence is not enough: Effects of emotional availability on infant exploration, *Developmental Psychology, 17,* 737-45

Strain, P.S. and Wiegernik, R. (1976) The effects of sociodramatic activities on social interaction among behaviourally disordered preschool children, *Journal of Special Education, 10,* 71-5

Ungerer, J. and Sigman, M. (1983) Symbolic play and language comprehension in autistic children, *Journal of the American Academy of Child Psychiatry* (in press)

Uzgiris, I.C. and Hunt, J. McV. (1975) *Assessment in infancy, ordinal scales of psychological development,* University of Illinois, Urbana

Werner, H. and Kaplan, B. (1963) *Symbol Formation,* Wiley, New York

Whittaker, C.A. (1980) A note on developmental trends in the symbolic play of hospitalized profoundly retarded children, *Journal of Child Psychology and Psychiatry, 21,* 253-61

6 PARENT-CLINICIAN INTERACTION IN THE REMEDIATION OF DISORDERED ARTICULATION

Ralph L. Shelton and Anita F. Johnson

Speech-language pathologists concerned with disordered articulation and other communication pathologies have several reasons for working with parents. Work with parents may be considered one means of preventing communication disorders. To the extent that delay in speech and language development reflects environmental influences, enhancement of parenting skills relative to communication may decrease the number of persons eventually requiring professional speech-language services. In cases where need for professional assistance is not prevented, the amount of professional therapy needed may be reduced through parent participation. Moreover, services provided to a child in the home or in the home and clinic may be more effective than those delivered in the clinic only.

This chapter reviews data and inferences about the role of parents in the treatment of children's articulation disorders. Much of the literature is written from a phonetic perspective and does not pertain to the use of phonological concepts to influence the child's sequencing of sounds in a mature pattern. Research is needed to formulate and test parent participation in therapy of a phonological nature. The literature cited focuses on the parent as an aide to the clinician. However, we also consider conceptual work that would have the clinician serve as a consultant to the parent. Some use is made of language literature as it provides a framework for consideration of articulation.

The importance that speech-language pathologists attribute to parent participation in therapy was evident in the results of a survey of speech-language clinics and training programmes conducted by Cartwright and Ruscello (1979). Eighty-nine per cent of the respondents indicated that parent involvement was an important part of their work. The survey indicated that parents are frequently called upon to work with their children to supplement work done by the clinician. Means of working with parents included conferences, parent observation of therapy, description of the child's performance in therapy, use of reference materials and parent discussion groups. Written reports to parents and parent observation of video-tapes of therapy were used infrequently.

Two kinds of evidence are often cited as justifying work with parents to facilitate speech-language development: (1) evidence that many parents often modify their language when talking to young children; and (2) evidence that children change their language in response to the environment. Schumaker and Sherman (1978) cited evidence that the language parents use with children is often simplified and redundant relative to that employed with more mature persons. Bloom and Lahey (1978) reviewed literature regarding caregiver input to children learning language and concluded that the speech most parents use with children is an excellent model for language learning. They note that it is simple, redundant and fluent, and is altered progressively as the child develops. Data supportive of these conclusions were published by Broen (1972), Snow (1972), Nelson (1973), Cramblit and Siegel (1977), and others.

Schumaker and Sherman (1978) also reviewed evidence that language development is influenced by learning variables such as imitation and reinforcement and that parents can utilise those variables to influence their children's speech. Hursh and Sherman (1973), for example, found that children's vocal behaviour could be controlled by rather simple procedures carried out by parents. They found that the frequency of a specific vocalisation was higher when parents modelled and praised it, than when they did not. Also, the frequency of a specific vocalisation was higher when modelling and praise were used in combination than when they were used separately.

Spradlin and Siegel (1982) discussed advantages and disadvantages of teaching language in the home. Generalisation is less of a problem when training is conducted in the home because children acquire skills in the environment in which they are used. Shortcomings of the home training include the possibility that few occasions for using appropriate models of language training may occur. For example, the television may compete with the child, or opportunities for language training may be pre-empted by the adults in the environment. If a child's speech is delayed, some alteration of parental practices is likely to be needed. As Goldstein and Lanyon (1971, p. 552) wrote, 'a child whose problems are based wholly or partly in the parents' own behaviors and attitudes is probably much less amenable to change by the parents'.

Spradlin and Siegel (1982) also discussed possible shortcomings of a clinical environment. A single clinician may work with the child in one room with the same stimuli used repeatedly. That which is taught in language programmes often does not resemble the language of normal social discourse. Training may involve repeating what has been said, naming objects, describing pictures, or making highly contrived requests. The verbal behaviour of the child is motivated by the teacher; it is not a natural response to the child's own needs or desires. Reinforcers used in the clinic, such as tokens, sweets, or even use of 'good' contingent upon certain responses is not likely to occur at home. Spradlin and Siegel suggest that training conducted in a professional setting be organised in a way that resembles the natural environment. Also, they acknowledge that there is little empirical information on home intervention programmes and they should be considered experimental.

The evidence cited above suggests that parents are capable of influencing children's speech and language development and that they use verbal behaviours that contribute to that development. Authors have used two conceptualisations of clinician-parent interaction in the facilitation of children's speech and language. In one, the clinician is considered to be a consultant to the parent. The clinician's task is to assist parents in establishing relationships with their children that encourage naturalistic development of language and speech. Clinicians following the second viewpoint employ parents as aides in teaching the child performances that are part of clinician-conducted therapy. First we shall consider the viewpoint that the clinician should serve as a consultant to the parent. This viewpoint has been directed to language rather than to articulation. It is cited here because it may be applicable to articulation and because it constitutes an alternative to the parent-as-aide construct.

The Speech Clinician as Consultant to the Parent

Hubbell (1981), writing about language — not articulation — disorder, discussed means of helping in the establishment of parent-child interactions from which language and speech evolve naturally. He questioned the practice of using parents as aides to extend the clinician's teaching. He wrote that clinicians who use parents as assistants take from the parents responsibility for effecting change in the child. He believes this practice is inconsistent with the parent's role as an agent for change in the child and may undercut that role. Hubbell's conceptualisation of speech-language delay is based on a transactional model in which the child's language is influenced by both the child's constitution and the environment. From this perspective, the child can influence the environment just as the environment influences the child. Thus feedback from the child influences parental speech; so to a degree children regulate the language models from which they learn. According to Hubbell the target of intervention for speech and language development should be transactions between the child and the environment. Such transactions are ways that family members regularly deal with one another. Parents may be helped to be more responsive to the child's efforts to communicate, and they may also be helped to provide suitable input to the child. Hubbell noted that home intervention should not be undertaken in the absence of specific goals and a favourable prognosis. Work done with parents should not require a great deal of time; however, time may lapse before the child begins to respond to changes in the parent's behaviour. The clinician should maintain contact with the parents during that period and should assess change in the child's communication.

Snyder and McLean (1976) and Snyder-McLean and McLean (1978) also discussed language acquisition in terms of interaction between the child and the environment. Through such interaction a child gains information about the world. The child then processes that information, thereby establishing a relationship between it and the linguistic code of his or her culture. Language development emerges as the child selectively attends to simple, comprehensible utterances and as adults provide appropriate feedback. Through interaction, mother and child establish joint reference; that is, they direct their attention to the same stimuli and come to use the same stimulus utterance associations.

A Committee of Inquiry in Great Britain used questionnaire and other study methods to investigate, among other things, the development of language (Bullock, 1975). The Committee concluded that many disadvantaged children lack experiences where someone listens to them, acknowledges their remarks and responds to their questions. Such children may come to school unprepared for conversations with an adult in which meanings are exchanged and questions are posed and answered. The Committee suggested such activities as a Mothers' Club, home visits by a liaison teacher, and formation of a mothers' nursery group for preschool children. The report also suggested that a parent can help prepare the young child for reading by holding him or her on the lap and reading aloud stories the child likes over and over again. The physical comfort and security combine with the fascination of the story to identify books as something which holds great pleasure.

We shall cite only three descriptive studies pertinent to the facilitation of children's speech and language and related variables through attention to parent-child transactions. A review of the literature on this topic is beyond the scope of this chapter. However, support is given to the ideas reviewed in this section by descriptive research reported by Levenstein (1970, 1971) and by Seitz and Marcus (1976). Levenstein developed a cognitive enrichment programme intended to help mothers to help their preschool children learn to learn. The families studied lived in suburban poverty areas. A Toy Demonstrator visited twice a week to demonstrate how the mother could increase daily interaction with her child through play. The visitor did not directly teach the child but rather demonstrated techniques that the mothers were free to use or not use. The children made intelligence quotient gains averaging 17 points.

Seitz and Marcus (1976) used observation and discussion to teach mothers to direct their speech to their children's activities. Parents were encouraged to use short, simple statements, restatement, interpretation or repetition of the child's remarks, and reinforcing utterances. Children were encouraged to accompany play with vocalisation. A case report was presented of a child who responded to this programme by increasing use of independent play and vocalisation and reducing use of negative and unresponsive behaviour.

This section has emphasised a role for the speech-language clinician in helping parents to establish relationships with their children that encourage child vocalisation and speech and language development. Next we shall consider ideas and empirical work wherein the parent serves as an assistant to the clinician helping to teach specific speech or language acts. Perhaps the two strategies can complement one another — especially if good parent-child transactions are established first.

Parent as Aide to the Clinician in Articulation Therapy

Employment of parents as aides in articulation therapy involves application of learning principles and knowledge — especially concerning reinforcement and generalisation. In this section, we shall consider reinforcement, knowledge of results and generalisation as they pertain to articulation therapy. Then we shall review empirical studies of services directed by clinicians but delivered by parents.

Reinforcement is sometimes defined in terms of stimuli that increase the frequency of responses that they follow. This after-the-fact definition was criticised as non-operational by Yates (1980). For purposes of articulation remediation, an informal concept of reinforcement is useful even though it does not take into account much of the study that has been directed to reinforcement as a theoretical abstraction. Stimuli directed to the child by the clinician both before and after articulatory responses can serve to motivate the child's continued participation in training and hence provide increased opportunities for learning through practice or problem-solving experiences. A variety of stimuli can serve to elicit desired responses and to provide information about performance to the child. The clinician learns to use these stimuli, which we consider to be reinforcing, in enhancing articulation improvement. The clinician may also teach parents to use the stimuli in articulation improvement.

Another learning variable, knowledge of results, is related to reinforcement. Yates (1980) provides a discussion of the distinction between the two. Knowledge of results involves an individual's use of information about his or her performance on a learning task. Like reinforcement, it is an abstraction. It may be sufficient to bring about wanted responses in articulation therapy. Van Houten (1980) differentiated between feedback systems and token-economies. The former use natural reinforcers that generalise well to new settings and require relatively little time, work or cost. Token-economies involve delivery of tokens for correct responses and exchange of the tokens for items valued by the learner. Van Houten suggested that only when feedback systems alone prove unsuccessful should additional reinforcers or a token-economy be considered. He stated that information feedback should be immediate and precise. Frequency of feedback is also important. He pointed out that research has shown that feedback should be kept positive to be optimally effective. The concepts of reinforcement and knowledge of results are important to parents who would participate in their children's articulation remediation. Parents' effectiveness as clinical aides may be influenced by how well they are taught to use reinforcement.

Generalisation learning is a particularly important topic in articulation therapy. Risley and Wolf (1968) defined generalisation as a phenomenon whereby appropriate behaviour occurs under conditions other than those in which the behaviour was originally learned. Parents can encourage their children to use newly-learned speech behaviours in appropriate contexts, and they can use events that occur naturally during the day to encourage speech generalisation to many situations. Mowrer (1971, 1982) listed management of speaking situations outside the clinic as an important instructional procedure to achieve generalisation. He concluded from his review (Mowrer, 1971) that parents, peers and teachers can be employed in ways that facilitate general-isation from clinical speech training. However, he noted that research was needed to test and develop procedures of this sort.

In recent years much research has been conducted relative to gener-alisation learning in the treatment of disordered articulation. McReynolds and Elbert (1982) cited evidence indicating that training directed to one sound often influences not only that sound but other sounds that share distinctive features with it. Sounds practised in one set of words may show generalisation to other words and to other activities such as reading and conversing. Similarly, training in the clinic often generalises to other settings. The enhancement of desired gener-alisation is of value to clinician and client. Unwanted generalisation can also occur; for example, learning of /s/ will sometimes generalise to /ʃ/ (Shelton, 1978).

In some studies, articulation learning in the clinic failed to generalise to non-clinic settings (Costello and Bosler, 1976). This sort of finding, in part, has motivated consideration of a role for parents in articulation learning. Conduct of training in a variety of settings is believed to be important to generalisation. Repetition at home of clinic drills and other activities might contribute to generalisation. Thoroughness of original learning may also facilitate generalisation.

Several investigations have employed parents as aides in the articul-ation treatment of their children. These studies may be sorted into three groups: (1) those in which, as part of traditional therapy, parents were given instruction about phonetics, articulation and therapy and then were instructed to teach articulation to their children; (2) those in which principles of operant conditioning and programmed instruction were employed to teach parents to conduct specific training procedures with their children; and (3) those in which parents were used as aides in the automatisation of articulation responses. The latter therapy was conducted within a perceptual-motor learning framework.

Parent as Aide in Traditional Therapy

Sommers, Shilling, Paul, Copetas, Bowser and McClintock (1959) studied the effects of training parents to help children with functional articulation defects. Thirty-six children and their parents were assigned to an experimental group and an equal number of children and parents were assigned to a control group. Children in both groups received artic-ulation therapy based on phonetic-placement principles, in the clinic four days weekly for a period of three and one-half weeks. Parents in the experimental group attended lecture-discussion periods during the first 30 minutes of their children's therapy sessions. Topics such as speech acquisition, speech problems, ear training, placement techniques and stimulating better speech at home were covered. The experimental group parents also observed their children's therapy after the discussion periods and met with the speech clinician for a short time to obtain specific advice and daily home assignments.

Control group parents were not encouraged to attend the lecture-discussion periods and did not attend their children's therapy sessions. No specific instructions were provided these parents by a clinician. Articulation improvement was measured by means of an articulation test that sampled ten consonants in the initial, medial and final positions of words. The authors concluded that children make more rapid gains with therapy when their parents receive training and participate in treatment. A later study (Sommers, 1962) confirmed the effectiveness of training mothers to assist in the correction of their children's misarticulations.

In another study, Sommers and his colleagues (Sommers, Furlong, Rhodes, Fichter, Bowser, Copetas and Saunders, 1964) studied the relationship between maternal attitudes and the amount of improvement in articulation that can be gained by training mothers to assist in articulation correction. The authors found that training was effective for both mothers with 'healthy' attitudes and for those with 'unhealthy' attitudes as measured by use of the Parental Attitude Research Instrument (Schaefer and Bell, undated).

Tufts and Holliday (1959) studied articulation therapy administered by parents to their preschool children. Forty-three children, whose articulation was rated 2, 3 or 4 on a five-point scale (wherein 1 represented unintelligible speech and 5 no articulation dysfunction), were randomly assigned to three groups: (1) a maturation group, (2) a professional therapy group, and (3) a parent therapy group. The ten children who received professional therapy worked together as a group for 46 sessions. Group members received training on sounds they misarticulated. Therapy included sound discrimination and production training, and social interaction in the clinic was also employed. The ten mothers in the parents' group met for an hour each week for 25 sessions and were provided information about correction of articulatory problems. Information was included about phonetics, articulatory placement techniques, ear training and production sequences from isolated sounds through syllables and words to connected speech. Discussion periods were conducted. The children received no professional therapy. Improvement was measured on the five-point scale cited above. The two treatment groups made statistically significantly greater gains than the maturation group. There was no significant difference in the gains achieved by the two treatment groups. The authors concluded that speech clinicians should consider using a portion of their time in training parents to assist in the treatment of their preschool children with moderately severe functional misarticulation.

The University of Pittsburgh (McWilliams, 1959) offered a non-credit course entitled Your Child's Speech Problems. The course was intended to provide parents with information about such topics as speech and child development, aetiologies of speech disorders, and professional services available to children with disordered communication. No attempt was made to offer clinical solutions to problems of parents' individual children who had not been professionally evaluated. The article describes the impact of the programme on individual parents. However, no data are reported. McWilliams concluded that the orientation of mothers to disordered speech is necessary if the children are to get the help they need.

McCroskey and Baird (1971) reported negative results in a study of parent participation in articulation therapy conducted as part of a school programme. As the authors point out, this study differed from many other studies involving parents in that children were assigned to groups that were or were not to receive parent assistance and then parent participation was solicited. If parents would not attend meetings at school, the clinicians went to the homes. The authors infer that effective parent participation in therapy is contingent upon the co-operation and ability of the parents.

A systematic parent programme was developed by Wing and Heimgartner (1973) to generalise articulatory skills to all speaking situations outside the clinic. The programme employed sequential steps varying in difficulty. It began with oral reading and progressed to oral reading and discussion, structured conversation, unstructured conversation within a set time span, and unstructured conversation within an extended time span. The children who participated in this study had been in public school speech programmes for at least two years but produced between 70 and 85 per cent of their target sounds incorrectly while reading to an unfamiliar examiner. Parents were trained to identify and record target speech sounds. Thereafter the clinician telephoned weekly or biweekly to monitor progress and answer questions.

Activities were written in detail and presented to child and parent during the training session. Each child was asked to work on the prescribed activity for ten minutes each day with the parent counting and recording target speech sound errors. The child began with the simplest level and proceeded to the next level only when there were no speech sound errors for three consecutive practice sessions. The child was made aware of goals, and the parent was instructed to reward the child for successful completion of each level if reward was thought to be necessary.

Results for six children in the pilot study indicated that children made no errors in an unstructured conversational situation after five to ten weeks and were ready for dismissal. An average of 40 ten-minute home practice sessions were required for completion of the programme. Parents did not use any tangible reinforcement during the programme. The parent training and weekly telephone calls required on the average less than a total of two hours of the clinician's time for each child. Similar results were obtained for 24 additional children.

Consideration of work with parents in traditional articulation therapy raises questions about how well clinicians communicate with parents. One means of working with parents is simply to communicate with them as they bring their children for evaluation and therapy. Eisenstadt (1972) interviewed parents of children receiving speech-language services. The parents expressed a number of concerns regarding the services they and their children received. They indicated that information and explanation were presented to them when they were preoccupied with other matters such as caring for another child who was present. Also, in providing explanation, the clinicians used terms unknown to the parents. The parents felt that they were not kept informed about progress and the likely duration of treatment and stated that instructions regarding work to be done at home after termination of formal therapy sometimes were not clear.

Parents as Aides in Operant-based Therapy

The Wing and Heimgartner study cited above reflects, in part, the influence of operant conditioning and its offspring programmed instruction on speech pathology. Other studies more clearly belong in that category. Several operant studies involving articulation training were reported in a book edited by Sloane and Macaulay (1968). Johnston (1968) presented a case study of a boy who was mentally retarded and emotionally disturbed. The boy's speech involved echolalia which included repeating words and phrases and mimicking the speech of others and of himself. His parents were instructed to elicit satisfactory speech at home through stimulation and reinforcement. The mother observed sessions in the laboratory and visited the child's classroom in order to learn how to use the same cues and directions at home that were used at school. The parents were to employ contingencies for the child's speech at home that were similar to those used in the laboratory. While data on the child's speech behaviour at home were not collected, the family reported his rate of verbalisations at home increased, and screaming occurred less frequently.

Sloane, Johnston and Harris (1968) developed a programme of small steps and immediate and concrete environmental consequences for shaping the speech of young children whose speech was absent, delayed or poorly articulated. A goal was to train mothers to do remedial work with their children at home. Training involved a progression of steps including simple nonverbal imitation, imitation of articulator placements for non-speech acts, and articulatory placement for speech sounds. Speech sounds and words were further developed through imitative shaping. Mothers were given verbal and written instructions that included information about training successive approximations of a desired behaviour and reinforcement. The parents demonstrated to the experimenters what they would do at home, and the experimenters gave suggestions and reinforcement to the parents. The parents returned to the laboratory to demonstrate and describe what they were doing at home and to obtain instructions. While no experimental control procedures were used, case reports presenting charts of performance on such variables as intelligible approximations and vocalisation indicated progress occurred.

Mowrer, Baker and Schutz (1968) described the development and validation of a programmed procedure for correction of frontal lisps. The programme became known as the /s/ pack. One goal of the study was to learn whether the programme could be administered successfully by someone other than a speech pathologist. The programme initially had three parts. The first part was intended to establish /s/ in monosyllabic words in sentences; the second part was to strengthen and maintain that which was learned in part 1. Part 3 was to extend production of /s/ to conversational speech. A teacher-volunteer not trained in speech pathology was successful in administering the programme. Of 20 subjects, 16 obtained perfect scores on a post-treatment test. The authors noted that the programme was useful with frontal lisps but not with omissions or substitutions other than the replacement of /s/ with /Ɵ/. Nor was the programme successful with children presenting open-bite.

A later study developed the /s/ pack further. Ryan (1971) employed a version of this programme that contained a fourth part. It was a home transfer programme to be administered by a parent or other 'transfer person'. No control group or procedure was used. The children studied improved their performance on a 30-item /s/ task from a pre-treatment mean of 2.2 to a post-treatment mean of 29.6. After treatment the mean percentage of correct /s/ sounds in a two-minute conversation was 77.1 per cent, with a standard deviation of 30.3. Of 18 children, eight produced all of their conversational /s/ sounds with their teeth in a closed-bite position; however, half of the children produced 89 per cent or fewer of their responses in that manner. Concern was expressed about the lack of carry-over in some subjects, and the question was raised whether the parents had reinforced the responses in conversation.

A number of additional operant studies have tried to help parents influence their children's articulation. A programme of articulation therapy for mothers was written by Carrier (1969, 1970). It was designed to teach any consonant sound which the child could successfully imitate. The mothers were given materials and instructions for presenting lessons. They were instructed to conduct two homework sessions per day; each session was 60 responses in length and required five to ten minutes. The programme consisted of 20 stimulus words, ten with the target sound in the initial position and ten in the final position. Lesson one called for the mother to present a picture stimulus and say the word, splitting it apart so that the target sound and the rest of the word were uttered with a pause between them. If the child correctly imitated the target phoneme, he or she was reinforced with verbal praise and a poker chip that could be exchanged for small toys or food items at the end of the session. If his or her response was incorrect, the mother withheld reinforcement and went on to the next picture. When the child achieved 20 consecutive correct responses, he or she progressed to lesson two. In lesson two the mother showed the same pictures and said the words without splitting them apart. In lesson three she showed the pictures but did not say the words. In lesson four she paired the picture with questions, objects or actions that required use of the target sound. In lesson five the picture was dropped and only questions, objects or actions containing the target sound were used as stimuli. In lesson six, objects were placed about the house and mother and child went from one to another naming them.

Ten children from four to seven years of age received lessons from their mothers. Ten other children served as control subjects. The mothers of the control children were instructed to tell their children when they made articulation errors on the assigned sound and to model for the children how to say their target sounds correctly. Subjects in the two groups were matched as closely as possible for age, score on an articulation test, and for assigned sound and cognate. The groups were compared for gains on their assigned sounds and the cognates of those sounds as measured by use of the Deep Test of Articulation (McDonald, 1964). Control subjects made no gains whereas experimental subjects made a mean gain of 19 items for the assigned sounds and 11 items for the cognates.

Fahey (1976) employed a programme similar to Carrier's to train parents to help their children correct misarticulations. Her training programme progressed from a one-word imitative level to a spontaneous sentence level. Fahey noted that her treatment and that of Carrier each employed a stimulus-shift hierarchy patterned after that described by McLean (1970). Stimuli included requests for imitation, naming and describing observed activities. Twenty-five children, ranging in age from 7 to 14 years, participated in the study, and 23 of them demonstrated sufficiently high levels of generalisation and maintenance at the conclusion of the programme that no further treatment was recommended. Dependent articulation measures included tests for the target sound and observation of the target sound in three-minute conversational samples. While no control group was employed, all subjects did make substantial articulation gains while receiving training over periods ranging from seven days to three months.

A version of Carrier's programme was also used by Costello and Bosler (1976) to investigate generalisation of correct articulation learned in the home to performance in other settings and on new stimulus words. Learning was studied in 20 training words and five nontraining words. The three young children who participated in the study showed articulation generalisation to nontreatment settings. However, outside the clinic setting the target sound /v/ was more frequently used correctly in training than in non-training words. The authors noted that articulation of a given sound differs in different contexts as a function of coarticulation and that the small corpus of training words employed in their study may not have provided needed motor practice with a variety of contexts. They suggested, then, that large numbers of stimulus words be included in articulation training programmes to provide experience with more contexts and to aid children in abstracting the target phoneme as a discriminative stimulus.

Additional evidence of successful home intervention through operant training was demonstrated in a programme structured to correct lisping of /s/ and /z/. It was conducted by a paraprofessional or parent acting as the child's instructor (Ueberle and Click, 1970). Nineteen elementary school children who could correctly imitate the /s/ phoneme participated in the study. Thirteen parents agreed to work with their own children, and the remaining six children were assigned to student aides. A three-lesson orientation was followed by daily ten minute lessons that required the child to make 104 responses. Each response involved the sequence of cue-response-feedback. At the end of the five week training programme, therapy effectiveness was evaluated though counts of responses in connected speech. Twelve children were considered to have had their speech problems corrected and were dismissed. Six children were considered to have had their problems corrected but were placed on observational dismissal. One child was not successful in the programme and was enrolled for additional therapy.

Goldstein and Lanyon (1971) taught parents of a ten-year-old autistic child to use modelling and reinforcement procedures to enhance their child's speech and language. The child possessed no intelligible speech at the beginning of the study. Training was directed to the intelligible production of words through imitation, to use of words for labelling, and to the use of simple phrases. The boy learned improved articulation of 83 words and some picture labelling and phrase usage.

Parents as Aides in the Automatisation of Articulation Responses

We have conducted two studies to assess the effectiveness of parent-administered activities for automatisation of articulatory responses (Shelton, Johnson and Arndt, 1975; Shelton, Johnson, Willis and Arndt, 1975). This work was based on a perceptual-motor information-processing model of articulation remediation. Acquisition and automatisation of responses are called for by the model (Shelton and McReynolds, 1979; Morris, McWilliams and Shelton, in press). The studies also reflect the influences of traditional speech pathology and of behaviourism. Parents in these studies monitored their children's speech for articulation of a target sound. Correct responses were to be rewarded with points that could be exchanged for prizes. The parent informed the child of misarticulations of target sounds and asked the child to repeat words in which a target sound was misarticulated so that the sound was corrected in the repetition.

The first study (Shelton, Johnson and Arndt, 1975) involved eight children who were able to imitate the target sound /s/ correctly. Three of the children had previously received speech therapy at school; the others had received no prior training. Training given to the children's mothers included auditory discrimination practice for identification of words which contained /s/ sounds, identification of the word position in which /s/ occurred, and discrimination between correct and incorrect /s/ productions. A short video-tape was used to demonstrate the procedure parents were to follow when working with their children at home.

During the first three days of the first week, parents also presented models to their children for imitation. The models consisted of words containing /s/ in the initial, medial or final position. On the fourth and fifth days, the parents listened to 20 /s/ sounds as they occurred in their children's description of television programmes, stories or events. The parents responded to the target sounds with reinforcement or requests for corrected repetitions as they later did for sounds occurring in spontaneous conversation. The remaining four weeks were devoted to the conversational monitoring described above in which the parent responded to approximately 40 /s/ sounds as they occurred in conversation each day.

The children were tested weekly for /s/ articulation in word imitation, talking and reading tasks. Statistically significant mean gains of seven and six items, respectively, were made on the talking and reading measures over the five-week period. The children's performance on the imitation tasks was high at the initiation of treatment, and no statistically significant gain was made on that task.

A similar study was carried out with ten preschool children (Shelton, Johnson, Willis and Arndt 1975). Before the home programme was started, the children were taught to produce a target speech sound (/s/, /l/, or /r/) in isolation and in words. The number of sessions required to teach the children such performance ranged from three to 13. Parent training and the parent monitoring task were similar to that described for the school-age children (Shelton, Johnson and Arndt, 1975). For these younger children, however, parents listened to approximately 30 target sounds in conversation each day. Again, they rewarded correct responses and asked for correct imitations of words articulated incorrectly. The parents were free to select a reward that they thought would be effective and to administer different rewards as they thought appropriate. Sweets and stickers were used most frequently. Performance on word imitation and talking measures showed statistically significant improvement over the five-week period. The data did not indicate, however, that usage of the target sound had been established on an automatic level.

Shelton, Johnson, Ruscello and Arndt (1978) investigated the effects of listening training on the speech of preschool children. The training was administered by the parents of the children and involved either sound discrimination training or story reading. Articulation of children assigned to these groups did not show significantly greater articulation improvement than did control group children. Additionally, there were no reliable differences in articulation improvement among the three groups in response to follow-up sound production training. While these particular procedures appeared to be ineffective in facilitating articulation improvement, it is possible that such training might have been effective if administered by speech pathologists. Also, another form of auditory training might have been more beneficial. The authors reported that some parents described reacting with anger and frustration to their children's performance on the listening tasks that were used. Advancement through training steps was not contingent upon a child's performance so that emphasis was placed on children's listening experiences rather than on correctness of their responses.

The research reviewed above, whether conceptualised in terms of traditional therapy, operant conditioning or perceptual-motor learning, suggests that parents can make important contributions to articulation therapy. Parent participation was effective in the motor learning studies involving speech production but not in the study involving auditory training.

Observations and Conclusions

Any consideration of parents as aides in articulation therapy must acknowledge that before parents can participate in therapy, they must meet other responsibilities to the child. Those responsibilities include loving and playing with the child and meeting the child's basic needs (Wulz, Hall and Klein, 1983).

We have reviewed information about parents as aides to the clinician in remediating disordered articulation and about the clinician as a consultant to parents in naturalistic facilitation of speech-language development. These ideas may supplement one another. Techniques directed to naturalistic facilitation of language development may be directed to articulation — especially to the carry-over or automatisation of articulatory skills. Schumaker and Sherman (1978), writing from a behavioural perspective, suggested that parents capitalise on teaching their children during what they termed incidental teaching episodes. These are situations that occur naturally in the home and in which children show an interest in interacting with their parents. Parents may take advantage of these situations as they occur to facilitate speech and language development. Daily structured lessons are not needed.

Schumaker and Sherman provided suggestions for conducting training of this sort. They would have parents talk to their children, teach imitation and prompt word and utterance usage. They noted that when talking, children are receptive to praise, questions and expansions. While parents often do these things spontaneously, they can find new opportunities for their use. We would extend this idea to articulation. Incidental teaching episodes can take the form of the parent stressing a target sound during a conversation with the child or commenting about or otherwise reinforcing spontaneous correct responses. When the child expresses interest in something, the parent may take the opportunity to call the child's attention to how the name of the object is said. It may be helpful to comment casually to the child from time to time about how much he or she has learned; You have learned ——— ; you are doing much better at ———.

Encouragement of constructive parent-child transactions and recommendations regarding things a parent might teach a child can be compatible in additional ways. Articulation treatment may be organised hierarchically, starting with establishment of a home environment that enhances speech-language development. Later articulatory skills may be taught to the child, and then the newly-learned skills may be carried to an automatic level. This is compatible with traditional methods of speech pathology treatment. Steps used with a particular child depend upon the child's needs.

Children who present poor development and usage of language and speech and poor relationships with their parents would appear to be good candidates for the services described by Hubbell (1981). Establishment of improved parent-child transactions may remove hindrances to maturation and thus facilitate speech and language development. For some children, this first step may be sufficient. Other children may need this step and other professional language and speech services. Still other children may not require the first step of improved parent-child transactions. Members of this group would include children whose language proficiency is appropriate to their ages and who readily use language to communicate. Their articulatory disorders are not accompanied by language delay. These children may benefit from parent administration of articulation tasks directed by the speech clinician.

Variables in addition to the nature of the child's communication disorder and the clinician's views about the parent's role in therapy will influence the clinician's interaction with parents in articulation therapy.

Other variables include the clinician's conceptualisation of disordered articulation and parent behaviours.

Misarticulation is conceptualised in different ways. McReynolds and Elbert (1982) described the relationship between the clinician's concept of disordered articulation and the recommended therapy. A model of disordered articulation that emphasises auditory discrimination calls for an emphasis on auditory discrimination in therapy. If disordered articulation is considered to reflect a deficit in sensorimotor skill or learning, then therapy is likely to emphasise speech production and its evaluation. Phonetic misarticulation and use of immature phonological patterns are related, and a child may receive phonetic and phonological therapies during the same session. The latter are often directed to elimination of phonological processes that are thought to simplify the child's sound pattern. One technique for accomplishing this is to present the child with speaking situations that require use of mature forms if communication is to be successful. We presume parents can be involved in work of this sort. Incidental teaching episodes may be useful to accomplish this goal.

A given clinical technique may be employed in more than one therapy model. Hence therapies of different theoretical origins may share techniques. Regardless, different tasks may be assigned to parents by clinicians following different therapy models. Each of the models cited in the previous paragraph is compatible with a distinction between response acquisition and response automatisation. The discrimination and sensorimotor models assume that the child who cannot already do so must learn to produce sounds in various contexts before they will be used in conversational speech. Phonological therapy, however, is usually directed to establishing use of sounds that the child can already produce. The desired end-point is the child's use of the sound pattern employed by adults in his or her community.

Little has been published about characteristics of parents as a variable in articulation therapy. Earlier we cited Sommers *et al.* (1964) to the effect that mothers with unhealthy attitudes as well as those with healthy attitudes were able to benefit from training provided to help them assist their children with articulation learning. Payne-Johnson (1982) observed that the USA is a multi-cultural community wherein family values differ. She indicated that adjustments in speech treatments may be necessary to accommodate family interests and wishes. Clinically we have observed that at least initially some parents don't listen to information provided by the clinician. Some repeatedly state opinions that they consider to be relevant to the child's articulation disorder. When the clinician asks for assistance, it is not uncommon for parents to ask if one of their other children can participate in therapy in their place. We do not recommend this practice unless care is taken to make sure that the sibling understands the task to be accomplished and can relate to the brother or sister in a helping way. Some parents agree to participate but do not do so, and many participate beautifully. Earlier we reported that some parents have expressed frustration at their children's performance in therapy tasks performed at home. This parental reaction requires an adjustment in therapy. It may be evidence of need for the clinician to provide assistance in parent-child transactions.

Evidence supportive of parental involvement in the treatment of their children's disordered articulation is sufficiently strong to encourage further research and cautious clinical application of the procedures that have been described and investigated. No one best plan for interacting with all parents in the treatment of disordered articulation is evident. With further research, this part of clinical practice may become more structured. In the meantime, the clinician's work with parents may be approached from a problem-solving viewpoint.

In our opinion, communication between parent and clinician is important whether the parent is to be involved in the therapy directly and extensively or indirectly and very litle. Clinicians should use language that is clear to parents, and communication should take place in a setting that allows both parties to attend to the conversation without distraction. Parents should be informed about the goals and nature of therapy, about the child's response to therapy, and about prognosis for future accomplishment and clinical needs. They should be given information about the nature of the child's articulation disorder; and if they are to participate in therapy, they should understand what is being done and why and also what is expected of them.

Regardless of whether parents are to assist in therapy directly, we encourage them to observe therapy sessions and to talk with us. Ten minutes of a 30-minute session are often devoted to talk with parents. Part of that time may be spent providing the parents with information. However, information may also be obtained from them. We often ask parents to tally correct and incorrect responses at home and to write down words with target sounds that are correctly articulated and those that are not. Parent observations and record keeping can be a useful source of information about a child's progress in therapy.

We have more experience in using parents to assist in the establishment of articulation responses in automatic speech than in having them assist with the acquisition of new articulatory responses. We think that teaching sound-production skills, when needed, is a task for the clinician. However, as sounds are established in words, they can be practised and used at home. Parental monitoring and reinforcement of correct conversational articulation at home appears to contribute to the solution of the carry-over problem.

If a parent is to serve as an aide in the administration of a task in articulation therapy, we provide the parents with training needed to understand and perform the task. This may involve perceptual training relative to the child's articulation. We demonstrate the activities and provide at least a written outline of the instructions that have been presented orally. Opportunities are given the parent to practise tasks under the clinician's observation. Somers (1980) found it effective to video-tape parents working with their children and to view and discuss the tapes with the parents privately. Whatever is done should not place pressure on child or parents. Indeed activities should be enjoyable for each party.

Acknowledgement

The authors wish to thank Dr Richard Curlee, Dr Rebecca McCauley and Dr Anne H.B. Putnam for their editorial contributions to this chapter.

References

Bloom, L. and Lahey, M. (1978) *Language Development and Language Disorders*, John Wiley, New York
Broen, P.D. (1972) The verbal environment of the language-learning child, *American Speech and Hearing Association Monograph, 17*, American Speech and Hearing Association, Washington, DC
Bullock, A. (1975) *A Language for Life*, HMSO, London
Carrier, J.K. (1969) *A Program of Articulation Therapy Administered by Mothers*, unpublished doctoral dissertation, University of Pittsburgh
———(1970) A program of articulation therapy administered by mothers, *Journal of Speech and Hearing Disorders, 35*, 344-53
Cartwright, L.R. and Ruscello, D.M. (1979) A survey on parent involvement practices in the speech clinic, *American Speech and Hearing Association, 21*, 275-9
Costello, J. and Bosler, S. (1976) Generalization and articulation instruction, *Journal of Speech and Hearing Disorders, 41*, 359-73
Cramblit, N.S. and Siegel, G.M. (1977) The verbal environment of a language-impaired child, *Journal of Speech and Hearing Disorders, 42*, 474-82

Eisenstadt, A.A. (1972) Weakness in clinical procedures — a parental evaluation, *American Speech and Hearing Association, 14*, 7-9

Fahey, V.K. (1976) A parent conducted program of articulation modification, *Human Communication, 1*, 19-27

Goldstein, S.B. and Lanyon, R.I. (1971) Parent-clinicians in the language training of an autistic child, *Journal of Speech and Hearing Disorders, 36*, 552-60

Hubbell, R.D. (1981) *Children's Language Disorders, An Integrated Approach*, Prentice-Hall, Englewood Cliffs, New Jersey

Hursh, D.E. and Sherman, J.A. (1973) The effects of parent-presented models and praise of the vocal behavior of their children, *Journal of Experimental Child Psychology, 15*, 328-39

Johnston, M.K. (1968) Echolalia and automatism in speech: a case report, in H.N. Sloane, Jr., and B.D. Macaulay (eds.), *Operant Procedures in Remedial Speech and Language Training*, Houghton Mifflin, New York

Levenstein, P. (1970) Cognitive growth in pre-schoolers through verbal interaction with mothers, *American Journal of Orthopsychiatry, 40*, 426-32

——(1971) Learning through (and from) mothers, *Childhood Education, 49*, 130-4

McDonald, E.T. (1964) *A Deep Test of Articulation*, Stanwix House, Pittsburgh

McCroskey, R.L. and Baird, V.G. (1971) Parent education in a public school program of speech therapy, *Journal of Speech and Hearing Disorders, 36*, 499-505

McLean, J.E. (1970) Extending stimulus control of phoneme articulation by operant techniques, in F.L. Giradeau and J.E. Spradlin (eds.), *A Functional Analysis Approach to Speech and Language, ASHA Monograph No. 14*, American Speech and Hearing Association, Washington, DC

——and Snyder-McLean, L.K. (1978) *A Transactional Approach to Early Language Training: Derivation of a Model System*, Charles E. Merrill, Columbus, Ohio

McReynolds, L.V. and Elbert, M.Fl (1982) Articulation disorders of unknown etiology and their remediation, in N.J. Lass, L.V. McReynolds, J.L. Northern and D.E. Yoder (eds.), *Speech, Language and Hearing, Volume 1, Normal Processes*, W.B. Saunders, Philadelphia

McWilliams, B.J. (1959) Adult education program for mothers of children with speech handicaps, *Journal of Speech and Hearing Research, 24*, 408-10

Morris, H.L., McWilliams, B.J. and Shelton, R.L. (in press) *Cleft Palate Speech*

Mowrer, D.E. (1971) Transfer of training in articulation therapy, *Journal of Speech and Hearing Disorders, 36*, 427-46

——(1982) *Methods of Modifying Speech Behaviors*, Charles E. Merrill, Columbus, Ohio

——Baker, R.L. and Schutz, R.E. (1968) Operant procedures in the control of speech articulation, in H.N. Sloan, Jr., and B.D. Macaulay (eds.), *Operant Procedures in Remedial Speech and Language Training*, Houghton Mifflin, New York

Nelson, K. (1973) Structure and strategy in learning to talk, *Monograph of the Society for Research in Child Development, 38* (Serial No. 149)

Payne-Johnson, J.S. (1982) Family intervention for inner-city populations, *American Speech and Hearing Association, 24*, 33-4

Risley, T. and Wolf, M. (1968) Establishing functional speech in echolalic speech, in H.N. Sloane, Jr., and B.D. Macaulay (eds.), *Operant Procedures in Remedial Speech and Language Training*, Houghton Mifflin, New York

Ryan, B.P. (1971) A study of the effectiveness of the s-pack program in the elimination of frontal lisping behavior in third-grade children, *Journal of Speech and Hearing Disorders, 36*, 390-6

Schaerfer, E.S. and Bell, R.Q. (undated) *Parental Attitude Research Instruments: Normative Data*, National Institute of Mental Health, Bethesda, Maryland

Schumaker, J.B. and Sherman, J.A. (1978) Parent as intervention agent, in R.L. Schiefelbusch (ed.), *Language Intervention Strategies*, University Park Press, Baltimore

Seitz, S. and Marcus, S. (1976) Mother-child interactions: a foundation for language development, *Exceptional Children, 42*, 445-9

Shelton, R.L. (1978) Services for individuals with speech disorders, in J.F. Kavanagh and W. Strange (eds.), *Speech and Language in the Laboratory, School, and Clinic*, MIT Press, Cambridge, Mass.

——and McReynolds, L.V. (1979) Functional articulation disorders: preliminaries to treatment, in N.J. Lass (ed.), *Speech and Language Advances in Basic Research and Practice, Volume 2*, Academic Press, New York

——Johnson, A.F. and Arndt, W.B. (1975) Monitoring and reinforcement by parents as a means of automating articulatory responses, *Perceptual and Motor Skills, 35*, 759-67

——Johnson, A.F., Ruscello, D.M. and Arndt, W.B. (1978) Assessment of parent-administered listening training for preschool children with articulation deficits, *Journal of Speech and Hearing Disorders, 43*, 242-54

——Johnson, A.F., Willis, V. and Arndt, W.B. (1975) Monitoring and reinforcement by parents as a means of automating articulatory responses II. Study of preschool children, *Perceptual and Motor Skills, 40*, 599-610

Sloane, H.N. and Macaulay, B.D. (eds.) (1968) *Operant Procedures in Remedial Speech and Language Training*, Houghton Mifflin, New York

——Johnston, M.K. and Harris, F.R. (1968) Remedial procedures for teaching verbal behavior to speech deficient or defective young children, in H.N. Sloane, Jr., and R.D. Macaulay (eds.), *Operant Procedures in Remedial Speech and Language Training*, Houghton Mifflin, New York

Snow, C.E. (1972) Mothers' speech to children learning language, *Child Development*, 43, 549-65

Snyder, L.K. and McLean, J.E. (1976) Deficient acquisition strategies: a proposed conceptual framework for analyzing severe language deficiency, *American Journal of Mental Disorders, 81*, 338-49

Snyder-McLean, L.K. and McLean, J.E. (1978) Verbal information gathering strategies: the child's use of language to acquire language, *Journal of Speech and Hearing Disorders, 43*, 306-25

Somers, M.N. (1980) The use of videotaping for self-evaluation in parent training, *American Annals of the Deaf, 125*, 729-30

Sommers, R.K., Shilling, S.P., Paul, C.D. Copetas, F.G., Bowser, D.C. and McClintock, C.J. (1959) Training parents of children with functional misarticulation, *Journal of Speech and Hearing Research, 2*, 258-65

——(1962) Factors in the effectiveness of mothers trained to aid in speech correction, *Journal of Speech and Hearing Disorders, 27*, 178-86

——Furlong, A.K., Rhodes, F.E., Fichter, G.R., Bowser, D.C., Copetas, F.G. and Saunders, Z.G. (1964) Effects of maternal attitudes upon improvement in articulation when mothers are trained to assist in speech correction, *Journal of Speech and Hearing Disorders, 29*, 126-32

Spradlin, J.E. and Siegel, G.M. (1982) Language training in natural and clinical environments, *Journal of Speech and Hearing Disorders, 47*, 2-6

Tufts, L.C. and Holliday, A.R. (1959) Effectiveness of trained parents as speech therapists, *Journal of Speech and Hearing Disorders, 24*, 395-401

Ueberle, J.K. and Click, M.J. (1970) Programmed contracts for /s/ and /z/ lisp correction by paraprofessionals, American Speech and Hearing Association Convention, New York

Van Houten, R. (1980) *Learning Through Feedback*, Human Sciences Press, New York

Wing, D.M. and Heimgartner, L.M. (1973) Articulation carryover procedure implemented by parents, *Language Speech and Hearing Services in Schools, 4*, 182-95

Wulz, S.V., Hall, M.K. and Klein, M.D. (1983) A home-centered instructional communication strategy for severely handicapped children, *Journal of Speech and Hearing Disorders, 48*, 2-10

Yates, A.J. (1980) *Biofeedback and the Modification of Behavior*, Plenum Press, New York

7 COMMUNICATION SUPPLEMENTS: PERSPECTIVES ON USAGE

Ena Davies

The child who does not talk presents a considerable challenge to parents responsible for care and professionals responsible for management. Attention is inevitably focused upon the child's failure to acquire language or develop functional speech, and remediation has logically been concentrated on improving expressive language. Whilst a speech-orientated approach might be appropriate in many instances, for other speechless children it may lead to an increased sense of failure when the goal of intelligible speech is not achieved. The situation may be further aggravated by the disappointment of parents and family and the frustration of therapists or teachers.

A communication-orientated approach is advocated by Silverman (1980) who suggests that the ultimate goal of therapy should be developing communicative skills to a level adequate to meet communicative needs. This rationale shifts the emphasis from an exclusive concentration on what the child cannot do to a perspective where residual abilities are effectively used to supplement speech.

In the course of language remediation there is not a clear dichotomy between a speech or communication-orientated approach. The approaches are not mutually exclusive and can and do co-exist in therapy. Intervention should be governed by the particular needs of the child and modified according to changes in communicative skills and behaviour. In this context supplements or augmentatives to speech have a valuable contribution to make as therapeutic tools, either as a support to speech for the child with impaired intelligibility or as a replacement to speech for the child with severe impairment. They can play an effective role as part of a behavioural approach to language acquisition and/or remediation (Premack and Premack, 1974; Deich and Hodges, 1977) or within a programme based on naturalistic considerations (Yoder, 1980).

Nonverbal behaviours exist as natural supplements to spoken output yet have often been neglected in therapy on the assumption that they may inhibit language development and suppress functional speech. These reservations appear unfounded. In fact the data show that the converse is true (Stokoe, 1976; Wilbur, 1979; Fristoe and Lloyd, 1977; Silverman, 1980): the introduction of supplementary means of communication is shown to support language development and facilitate expressive speech. If, as is suggested (Mehrabian, 1972), spoken output constitutes only 35 per cent of the communication process, remediation programmes which disregard the residual 65 per cent demonstrate a remarkable degree of tunnel vision.

Potential Users

Children with hearing impairment are perhaps the most easily identifiable users of speech supplements. Manual signing has long been established as a 'natural language' for communication amongst deaf people. However, the controversy still rages between those educators who maintain an oral approach to facilitate integration into a hearing environment, and those who support sign language to augment poor verbal abilities. However, Wilbur (1979) suggests that although the data do not argue convincingly in favour of signed English forms as opposed to American Sign Language, they do argue that signs in any form are better than no signs at all. Not even in this well-researched area is there agreement on whether supplements should be taught and, if they are, which systems should be chosen and how they should be taught. These questions have obvious implications for other potential users and systems.

The *mentally retarded* child may have little understanding of the language of the environment, but provided with an appropriate means of controlling that environment may develop some cognitive, educational and social skills. The assumption that mentally retarded children have little or nothing to communicate may become a self-fulfilling prophesy when no provision is made for their communicative needs. More recently non-speech systems have been increasingly explored as part of therapeutic or educational programmes for *autistic* children and *elective mutes* where previously little or no provision had been made (Kiernan, 1983).

Therapy for the *dysphasic* child may also include nonverbal systems. Code and Müller (1983) identify six perspectives for consideration in adult aphasia therapy — linguistic, nonverbal, neuropsychological, psychosocial, behavioural and evaluative. These perspectives are equally worthy of consideration in the management of childhood dysphasia. The introduction of a nonverbal system may have linguistic implications, may affect neural reorganisation, and has already been shown to have psychosocial and behavioural benefits (Fristoe and Lloyd, 1977).

The *dysarthric* child often has well-developed receptive language - but the motor disorders of respiration, phonation, articulation, resonance and prosody which are features of dysarthria disrupt expressive speech, often to the point of complete unintelligibility. Therapeutic intervention is often frustrated by the severity of the disorder, and the introduction of a supplement or an augmentative to support poor functional speech has, in the words of one cerebral palsied teenager, bridged the gap for 'the poor paralysed, tongue-tied person, who despite all ghoulish appearances happens to be callously crucified by a mocking normal intelligence' (Nolan, 1981).

Dyspraxia interferes with volitional control over articulation and prosody, in the absence of incoordination or paralysis. Rosenbek, Collins and Wertz (1976) identifies three major roles the clinician may fulfil in the management of apraxia — prophylactic, facilitatory and reorganisational. In each of these spheres non-speech systems may have a contributory part to play. Children with *cranio-facial abnormalities* may also benefit from a supplementary system as a short-term procedure, a support to be dispensed with once the child communicates effectively through speech.

Systems in Use

The evaluation of supplementary systems as therapeutic tools is still in its infancy. The efficacy of specific systems and the rationale for selection is ripe for investigation. A survey of the *use* of non-speech systems in special education in the UK has been undertaken by Kiernan, Reid and Jones (1979, 1982). The survey identifies the more frequently used systems, many of which were developed to fulfil a specific need, but have become adopted, or adapted, to meet the needs of other 'non-communicators'.

British Sign Language

Probably the oldest established 'natural' language for the deaf in Britain and developed by deaf people for their own use. It is an immediate and direct means of communicating using manual signs supplemented by alphabetic finger spelling. Its prime advantage is that it is unaided, dependent only on adequate hand control and visual and kinaesthetic retention of signs. Criticism can be levied at its apparent lack of grammatical structure — an issue worthy of further investigation. Along with other manual sign systems both user and receiver need to understand the code for effective two-way communication.

Makaton Vocabulary (Walker, 1976a and b)

A developmental language programme utilising British Sign Language as an expressive medium. The scheme devised by Walker and colleagues for mentally handicapped residents at Botleys Park Hospital, Chertsey, is now extensively used throughout the UK. (See Chapter 8 for a critical discussion of this approach.)

Paget-Gorman Systematic Sign System

Devised by Paget and Gorman as a conceptually-based manual sign system paralleling spoken English. It allows for a precise interpretation of the spoken word governed by grammatical rules. The creators' prime motivation was to improve the linguistic abilities of deaf children, but this system has been demonstrated to have benefits for other speechless or language-impaired children (Craig 1978; Crystal and Craig, 1973).

Cued Speech

Probably more speech orientated than any of the other supplements referenced in this chapter. A set of eight hand shapes 'cue' the position for articulation of vowels and consonants to clarify speech for the deaf child and improve their spoken output. The system was developed by Cornett at Gallaudet College, USA, in 1966 to facilitate lip reading and improve expressive speech (Cornett, 1967; Dixon, 1978).

Amer-Ind

This is probably the oldest gestural code in existence, having been used by the nomadic tribes of American Indians to overcome the barriers of spoken language. Pantomimic gestures are easily recognised and interpreted by the receiver. The use of this gestural communication code for speechless patients has been pioneered by Skelly (1979).

Blissymbolics Communication

A conceptually-based visual language. Pictographic, ideographic and abstract symbols are presented on a portable display. The written word appears with the symbol for ease of interpretation by the receiver and as visual reinforcement for the user. Symbolic systems are used primarily by those with physical handicap, either as a communication aid or educational tool (Silverman, McNaughton and Kates, 1978; Hehner, 1980; McDonald, 1980).

Picture Boards

Picture boards utilising pictorial representations have long been used to provide an expressive medium for the physically handicapped, non-reading child (McDonald and Schultz, 1973). The restriction on vocabulary is obvious — concrete representations are constrained by the number of pictures which can be displayed within arm's reach or indicated by visual gaze. The choice of vocabulary is also limited and often determined by the perspective of the professional or caregiver, rather than a direct consideration of the needs of the user. The inclusion of basic needs like food, drink and toilet are appropriate to bring about limited control of the immediate environment, but these items are singularly unmotivating to a potential user whose basic needs are met routinely.

Recent technological advances have utilised existing visual therapeutic approaches with aids geared towards specific developmental levels — pictorial, symbolic, alpha-numeric or word-based. These new tools can be used to support residual skills (e.g. Cannon Communicator for a child with good spelling ability and adequate hand function; 'Splink' as a word-based communication aid linked to television display; or aids incorporating synthetic speech such as Handivoice or Blisstalk). The full potential of these technological advances has yet to be realised. Silverman's (1980) prediction that no child, however severely handicapped, should be without some means of communication, is becoming an increasing reality as expertise develops in the production and provision of these aids.

Considerations on 'Accessing'

Methods of accessing or operating these devices depend on the user's physical abilities. Direct accessing by finger, fist or foot may be possible for some physically handicapped children. Others may have to depend on eye-pointing as their sole means of direct indication. For the more severely handicapped, 'indirect' accessing techniques may be necessary, using switches adapted for their particular needs. Direct accessing is obviously preferable as an immediate motor response may have more of a facilitatory effect on speech than the indirect techniques which use switches as an intermediary stage in the communication output. Indirect accessing also demands higher cognitive ability to perform the task. The importance of the multidisciplinary approach is essential to match the aid to the child and ensure its effective use. Many expensive aids gather dust in cupboards because the basic selection and matching procedures have been disregarded. (Vanderheiden and Grilley, 1975; Vanderheiden, 1981). The selection of an appropriate communication aid may depend on the clinician, but the operation of the aid will depend on positioning, seating and accessing techniques, involving the expertise of physiotherapists, occupational therapists and bio-engineers.

Although Yoder (1980) recommends a comprehensive assessment procedure prior to the selection of an aid or supplement, this is vastly different from that which exists in practice. Kiernan (1977) suggests that one of the prime considerations in determining the choice of a sign *or* symbol system appears to be that of upper limb function — those with good hand control are assigned to a 'signing' programme whereas those with poor co-ordination are assigned to a visual or symbolic system. An economic factor to take into consideration is that signing systems are unaided, and, apart from training personnel, incur no revenue consequences!

Ideally, assessment procedures taking into consideration psycholinguistic skills, cognitive abilities, motor skills, communication needs, social-emotional level and relevant background history are necessary (Yoder, 1980). Additional considerations are age, auditory and visual skills, the present means of communication and the environment in which the child lives. Time and support from parents and caregivers are essential to the effective implementation of any supplementary system.

There can be no prescription of specific systems or aids for specific disorders. As with any other therapeutic intervention each child has to be considered individually rather than labelled as 'dysphasic', 'mentally retarded' or 'dysarthric'. Until the processes involved in language acquisition in 'normal' children are more fully understood, how much further away is the solution for those who have not and cannot develop those skills? Do these children mirror normal developmental stages when provided with a communicative outlet, or does the pathological disorder mitigate against using developmental norms? In many instances speech-handicapped children are being provided with a visual system to supplement poor or absent speech. Vygotsky (1962) suggests a time lag of 6-7 years between the acquisition of linguistic skills in normal children and their expression in written form. The speechless child often has to rely exclusively on visual output as the expressive mode, whereas the normal child has the advantage of auditory-vocal feedback as a monitoring process. The author has seen many instances where cerebral palsied children, assessed on standardised language tests as 'within normal limits', when presented with a communication outlet, demonstrate severe syntactical problems and bizarre spelling errors. How much impact does the lack of auditory-vocal feedback have on the acquisition of linguistic skills and cognitive development? These questions have important implications in terms of *what* systems are taught and *how* they are taught.

Whilst freedom of choice in the selection of systems is essential, the present *ad hoc* approach to non-speech systems is a cause for concern. The criteria for selecting systems is as idiosyncratic as the criteria used (or not used!) to match the system to the child. Popularity of systems may be related to fashionable trends in education or therapy, the ability of the system's proponents to 'sell' the approach, the potential market of users, ease of learning and teaching, and the cost of implementing programmes, together with support and maintenance to ensure continuity. The emotive reaction generated by the success of a particular system is a powerful motivator. The mere fact that a system 'works' may be adequate reward for the speechless child and the therapist or teacher. However, it leaves unanswered the two important questions of *how* and *why* certain systems work.

It is hardly surprising, therfore, that in the UK certain Local Education Authorities have adopted a policy of single-system usage within a circumscribed area (Kiernan, 1983). This 'core curriculum' approach appears a logical course to steer through the bewildering multiplicity of systems available. However, this is a policy fraught with difficulties for those children for whom the chosen system is not appropriate.

Acceptability

Acceptability of communication supplements may present more of an obstacle to parents and professionals than to the potential user. In a preliminary report on parental attitudes towards Blissymbolics (Tew, Davies and Fletcher, 1980) the early reservations of parents regarding the idea of such an abnormal form of communication were overcome by the demonstrable improvement in communicative ability. Amongst those parents expressing qualified support (66.7 per cent) to this supplementary means of communication, fathers expressed more doubts than mothers, who appeared to have a more realistic attitude towards their child's handicap. Those parents who were neutral in their response (9.3 per cent) were either indifferent to their child's problem or felt that the responsibility for meeting the child's communicative needs rested with the school. Others regarded the introduction as yet another unreliable idea or as a short-term crutch only. A small percentage (7.4 per cent were unfavourable in their attitude. Whether these comments can be applied to other systems is too sweeping a generalisation but it would appear likely that parental attitudes towards any supplementary communication system would show a similar spread of opinion. From informal contact with care staff in residential centres both in the UK and the USA, the author has found that they also expressed reservations for very different reasons. Children, formally non-communicators, begin to assert their rights once given a means of expression. This places more demands on time for staff, who previously could attend to basic routine without interruption! The transformation from 'noncommunicator' to 'communicator' also has social implications for care staff and others within the child's environment. The speechless child is knowingly or unknowingly a silent witness to all the events in the environment, safe in the knowledge that these events will remain secret. The speechless child with a communication outlet has a powerful tool at his or her disposal!

Acceptability of a supplement to speech for the therapist or teacher may need an adjustment in attitude. The term 'alternative' to speech which crept into the vocabulary about ten years ago, suggests the failure that many professionals experience when they cannot meet their goals on behalf of the child. Supplements or augmentatives to speech are regarded as a 'last ditch resort' to be used only when all else has failed. This negative attitude denies the child the possibility of communicating at an earlier age, with the possible accrued advantage of stimulating language and verbalisation. An indictment against this attitude was expressed to the author by a young cerebral palsied woman (using her electronic aid): 'For ten years I tried to talk; they say I must try harder; I cannot talk.' Conversely, the attitude which regards the introduction of a supplement as an end in itself, denies the child the essential support from the initial introduction of the system to the point of independent communication. Consideration may also be given to the transition from one system to another should the need arise, for example from sign to symbol to electronic aid. Nor need the systems be mutually exclusive: signing and visual systems are used in conjunction with each other to provide a constant visual referent for a transitory sign system, assisting both communicator and receiver (MacDonald, 1984).

From the user's perspective acceptability may depend on very different criteria. Speed of communication is substantially reduced in any mode other than speech. Rate is essential to hold the attention of one's audience. Frustration and irritation creep in on the part of the listener, as the rate decreases. The cosmetic appearance of an aid or supplementary system is also important to the user who seeks to be as unobtrusive as possible. Size and portability of an aid or supplement are features to consider for the ambulant child. Perhaps the most important consideration for the user is how others perceive him or her and in that respect the more 'normal' the system the more acceptable it will be.

Implementation

Whilst it may be possible to define the systems and the potential users, the manner in which these systems are taught may be widely disparate. They may be implemented in programmes governed by developmental, behavioural or naturalistic considerations. It may be argued that the only natural supplements to speech are those of spontaneous gestures, facial expressions, body movements and sounds (Kylén, 1982). In some programmes these criteria are strictly observed. As these natural reactions do not constitute 'true' language what of the child with good receptive language yet who is deprived of an expressive medium other than these natural reactions? The onus of responsibility rests with the 'receiver' of the 'dialogue' to interpret these reactions using the tedious yes/no 'twenty questions' routine. A naturalistic approach would be self limiting if it utilised only residual behaviour without some enhancement.

Supplementary systems have been successfully implemented in programmes using behavioural techniques (Silverman, 1976). However, because of the interdependence between the technique and the system it is difficult to see whether it is the supplement *or* the technique which is effective. Many programmes based on developmental 'norms' may be strongly influenced by behavioural techniques. Therapists and teachers inevitably seek to modify the communicative behaviour of the children in their care and knowingly, or unknowingly, reinforce 'acceptable' attempts at communication. Initially, children are rewarded for any communicative response and thrive on the attention received. They may even elaborate their ideas in order to hold that attention. Another feature observed by the author following the introduction of a speech supplement to teenage children with good receptive language, was the pleasure derived from the use of expletives and socially unacceptable comments! This is reminiscent of the 3-4-year-old who revels in the feigned shock of the adults in the environment when a new 'rude' word is added to the vocabulary. Although one would not wish to inhibit the output of children with a newly acquired communication skill there may need to be some modification to ensure that once fluent communication is established some guidelines for social acceptability are observed, particularly in those instances where recording of output is undertaken, or a hard-copy printout is available as a permanent record.

The introduction of a non-speech system may be dictated by the clinician as an aid to communication or by the teacher as an educational tool. Parents too are often the initiators in an attempt to improve their interaction with their speechless child. The type of programme may therefore be governed by the person responsible for the introduction of the supplement. Whoever is responsible for the programme, it is essential for the child's benefit that *all* concerned become involved in order to expand and generalise use in the environment. Perhaps this is even more essential for 'signing' programmes than for those systems which can be more easily understood.

The primary goal of the instructor, regardless of the system, should be to meet the child's communicative needs. The introduction of the supplement may be to provide an expressive medium for those with good receptive language; to contribute towards language development in those with comprehension difficulties; or to provide a basic means of expression for those with limited ability (Silverman et al., 1978).

Therefore it is obviously essential that whoever is responsible for the choice of system takes into consideration the following factors.

(i) The child's desire to communicate is clearly of prime importance. This desire to communicate has often been extinguished in those whose attempts to make themselves understood have met with constant failure. Equally, the constant repetition of single items on a display does not constitute conversation. The desire to communicate may be rekindled by providing the child with something meaningful to communicate in an environment conducive to communication.

(ii) The means of communication currently used by the child need careful consideration. If 'natural' can this be expanded for more effective communication? If using a supplementary system, is the use appropriate and acceptable to the child and his or her environment? There are instances where children introduced to a system are deprived of that means of communication when transferred to another school or centre where the system is not known or used. For the fluent user this is the equivalent of being condemned to silence.

(iii) The child's psycholinguistic skills and how they have been assessed is another important factor. Is comprehension of language adequate to allow for the introduction of a symbolic or orthographic system, or is comprehension impaired to the extent that basic communication only may be possible? What degree of functional speech is available to the child? Expressive language may be minimal with a vast discrepancy between receptive and expressive skills. However, the child with a degree of functional speech, however unintelligible, may prove more resistant to using a supplement than the child with no speech at all. The tools for assessment are not specific to speechless children but are often used to provide qualitative and quantitative information prior to implementing a non-speech system. The child's cognitive skills in relation to educational level, learning rate, short- and long-term memory, and ability to recall and use are also essential features in learning and using any system effectively.

(iv) Motor skills, as suggested earlier (Kiernan, 1977), have often been considered as prime factors in determining the choice between sign or symbol programme. Gross motor skills and fine motor skills have implications in terms of accessing: an ambulatory child may reject a system that involves carrying a device, whereas the wheelchair-bound child may find portability less of a problem. Auditory and visual acuity need to be established before introducing aids, given the high degree of visual activity and perception many demand. Auditory feedback is also a valuable reinforcement and equally important to consider.

(v) The child's communication needs are important considerations at the outset to help determine vocabulary selection, school needs, social interaction, peer communication and family responses. The child's age will also have a bearing on specific communicative needs and will influence vocabulary choice.

(vi) Relevant background information relating to educational, medical and previous therapy will be useful for the instructor. The disruption of voluntary movement by the persistence of primitive reflexes is a major factor to consider in the selection of supplements and accessing, especially for the cerebral palsied child.

The preceding considerations are not exhaustive but are of considerable importance when it comes to evaluating specific systems in relation to specific children.

The manner in which the supplements are taught is also crucial. Teaching is often undertaken by individual withdrawal from the class or group (Kiernan, 1983) and often by the speech therapist responsible for implementing the communication supplement. Teachers, however, appear to teach supplements within the group context. There are arguments for and against both approaches. Children taught by speech therapists on a one-to-one basis may find the early acquisition of vocabulary easier in the confines of a closed environment. The analysis and selection of signs or symbols appropriate for the individual child may be made on the basis of psycholinguistic skills as part of a communication-based approach; whereas, in the classroom situation the objective may be more educationally biased. Vocabulary selection is sometimes determined by the child's educational needs and the possible acquisition of reading skills through the medium of a supplementary system rather than on the basis of the child's social needs.

The advantage of individual withdrawal lies in the exclusive concentration on user-specific vocabulary reinforced by behavioural techniques. In most instances supplements are taught through a multi-sensory approach, reinforced by auditory or visual feedback, or some token reward. The only supplement in which a multi-sensory approach is not advocated is that of Amer-Ind. Skelly (1979) suggests that at a pre-symbolic level a multi-sensory approach is likely to confuse and conflict, and a single-channel input and output is recommended. However, within the classroom or social setting there is more opportunity for spontaneous use with peers or other adults. The opportunity for interaction may develop more effective use of acquired communication skills.

The involvement of parents in the selection of system, teaching and vocabulary choice has not been fully explored. In residential schools it is not always possible to have active participation by parents because of constraints of distance and time. However, training courses for teaching supplementary systems encourage parent participation, and in some areas parent groups have been established to provide mutual support.

Both professionals and parents are responsible for the generalisation of system use from the confines of the speech therapy situation or the classroom to home and community. The flow of information needs to be two-way from school to home, reporting on events which may assist in understanding the child's first attempts at communicating by a supplementary means. The joy at conveying a message which is understood by the recipient may be justification enough for the introduction of supplements. However, recording of data is vital in the attempt to evaluate the use and efficiency of systems. Until this evidence is available there can be no clear guidelines for selection or teaching. There is little information to support one system rather than another, and even less evidence to support one specific approach to teaching supplementary communication systems rather than another.

In conclusion it is suggested that for those responsible for the implementation and teaching of systems there is an obvious need to develop systematic behavioural approaches: however for the speechless child, the prospect is more optimistic and as Silverman (1980) argues it would be difficult to conceive of a child or adult who is so severely handicapped there would be no non-speech system that he or she could use.

References

Code, C. and Müller, D.J. (1983) *Aphasia Therapy*, Edward Arnold, London

Cornett, C. (1967) 'In answer to Dr. Moores', *American Annals of the Deaf, 114*, 27-9

Craig, E. (1978) Introducing the Paget-Gorman Sign System, in T. Tebbs (ed.), *Ways and Means*, Globe Education, Basingstoke

Crystal, D. and Craig, E. (1973) Contrived Sign Language, in I. Schlesinger and L. Namir, (eds.), *Current Trends in the Study of Signed Language for the Deaf*, Academic Press, New York

Deich, R.F. and Hodges, P.M. (1977) *Language Without Speech*, Souvenir Press, London

Dixon, J.P. (1978) Cued Speech, in T. Tebbs (ed.), *Ways and Means*, Globe Education, Basingstoke

Fristoe, M. and Lloyd, L.L. (1977) Manual communication for the retarded: A resource list, *Mental Retardation, 15*, 18-21

Hehner, B. (1980) *Blissymbolics for Use*, Blissymbolics Communication Institute, Toronto, Canada

Kiernan, C.C. (1977) Alternatives to speech; A review of research on manual and other forms of communication with the mentally handicapped, *British Journal of Mental Subnormality, 23*, 6-28

——(1983) The use of non-vocal communication techniques with autistic individuals, *Journal of Child Psychology and Psychiatry 24*, 339-75

——Reid, B.D. and Jones, L.M. (1979) *Survey of the use of Signing and Symbol Systems*, Thomas Coram Research Unit, University of London, Institute of Education

——Reid, B.D. and Jones, L.M., (1982) *Signs and Symbols: Use of Non-Vocal Communication Systems*, University of London, Institute of Education, Studies in Education, No. 11, Heinemann, London

Kylén, G. (1982) Non-verbal communication and mental handicap, in *Distech. 1982*, Spastics Society, London

MacDonald, A. (1984) Blissymbolics and manual signing, Proceedings of XIX Congress of the International Association of Logopaedics and Phoniatrics (in press)

McDonald, E.T. (1980) *Teaching and Using Blissymbolics*, Blisssymbolics Communication Institute, Toronto, Canada

McDonald, E.T. and Schultz, A.R. (1973) Communication boards for cerebral palsied children, *Journal of Speech and Hearing Disorders, 38*, 73-88

Mehrabian, A. (1972) *Non-Verbal Communication*, University of Chicago Press,

Chicago

Nolan, C. (1981) Bridging the gap, in *Distech. 1981*, Spastics Society, London

Premack, D. and Premack, A.J. (1974) Teaching visual language to apes and language deficient persons, in R.L. Schiefelbusch and L.L. Lloyd (eds.), *Language Perspectives – Acquisition, Retardation, and Intervention*, University Park Press, Baltimore

Rosenbek, J.C. Collins, M. and Wertz, R.T. (1976) Intersystemic reorganisation for apraxia of speech in adults, *51st Annual American Speech and Hearing Association Meeting*, Houston, Texas

Silverman, F.H. (1980) *Communication for the Speechless*, Prentice-Hall, Englewood Cliffs, New Jersey

Silverman, H. (1976) The educational application of the Ontario crippled Children's Centre symbol communication program for other groups of exceptional children, Report Ontario Crippled Children's Centre, Toronto, Canada

——McNaughton, S. and Kates, B. (1978) *Handbook of Blissymbolics*, Blissymbolics Communication Institute, Toronto, Canada

Skelly, M. (1979) *Amer-Ind Gestural Code: Based on Universal American Indian Hand Talk*, Elsevier, New York

Stokoe, W.C. (1976) The study and use of sign language, in R.L. Schiefelbusch (ed.), *Nonspeech Language and Communication; Analysis and Intervention*, University Park Press, Baltimore

Tew, B., Davies, E. and Fletcher, P. (1980) Parental Attitudes towards Blissymbolics, *College of Speech Therapists Bulletin, 334*, 8-10

Vanderheiden, G.C. (1981) Critical factors in the selection of augmentative communication techniques for severely handicapped people, in *Distech. 1981*, Spastics Society, London

—— and Grilley, K. (1975) *Non-vocal Communication Techniques and Aids for the severely Physically Handicapped*, University Park Press, Baltimore

Vygotsky, L.S. (1962) *Thought and Language*, MIT Press, Cambridge, Mass.

Walker, M. (1976a) *The Makaton Vocabulary* (revised edition) Royal Association in Aid of Deaf and Dumb, London

——(1976b) *Language programmes for use with the Revised Makaton Vocabulary*, private publication, Chertsey, Surrey

Wilbur, R.B. (1979) *American Sign Language and Sign Systems*, University Park Press, Baltimore

Yoder, D.E. (1980) Communication systems for non-speech children, *New Directions for Exceptional Children, 2*, 63-78

SECTION III: CRITICAL CONSIDERATIONS

The final section of this book examines from a more critical perspective, some of the important issues which have been raised. In the opening chapter Kiernan suggests some criteria which can be used for evaluating remedial language programmes. These criteria are then used to evaluate four programmes to illustrate how they can be applied and special emphasis is given to the Makaton programme because of its widespread usage in the UK. Kiernan's discussion leads him to question whether it is actually possible to develop an adequate language programme. He suggests instead that it might be better if there were more dialogue between researchers and practitioners in formulating language remediation strategies.

In the next chapter Howlin presents an extensive review of published research on parents as therapists. She outlines the effects of parents' speech to children, and although she suggests that there is no causal link between language input and language development, it is concluded that parental involvement in language intervention programmes would seem to be important for success. This chapter emphasises the importance of evaluating the efficacy of parental involvement and a large number of studies are reported. The importance of individual differences is stressed ·and the need to collect more data on the type of children for whom language training works is discussed. In conclusion, Howlin reiterates the need to follow the basic requirements of experimental design in evaluating parental contributions to language remediation.

The final chapter in this section and the book, questions the whole basis for teaching children to develop language. Harris suggests the assumption that the sequence of language abilities which spontaneously develop in normal children can be established in language-disordered children, lacks firm empirical support. From a detailed analysis of the processes of 'development' and 'teaching', he illustrates the problems inherent in trying to teach children to develop language. His view is that the aim of intervention should be to facilitate developmental processes in which special emphasis is given to situational variables. The need for more research concerning the nature of social interaction between language-disordered children and their caretakers is discussed. In raising these important questions, Harris illustrates the need to adopt a *critical* yet *constructive* approach in implementing language remediation with children. It is hoped that this volume has gone some way towards achieving this balance in discussing behavioural and naturalistic approaches.

8 LANGUAGE REMEDIATION PROGRAMMES: A REVIEW

Chris Kiernan

In this chapter I will discuss language remediation programmes as developed for use with the severely mentally handicapped. During the last two decades we have seen an increasing effort to relate theory to practice in language remediation and to spread 'good practice' through the publication of an increasing number of texts. Part of this effort has yielded a number of published or mimeographed guides to teaching in which a variety of steps are laid out through which the practitioner is recommended to take the student in order to teach language skills.

The first part of the chapter will briefly allude to studies which have been used as the foundations for language programming. The conclusion, which will be drawn from this discussion is that the studies, although of substantial practical value, all reflect an absence of unequivocal guidance which can act as a sure foundation for a programme.

In the next section I will put forward several criteria for the evaluation of remedial language programmes and will then examine a few important or highly considered programmes against these criteria. It will be shown that none of the programmes succeed in meeting all of the requirements for a good programme. Failure sometimes occurs because programmes are out of date conceptually or because their proponents simply fail to provide any evidence which suggests that they work.

In conclusion it will be argued that the development and publication of language remediation programmes is a difficult undertaking which is almost certain to fail, especially at a time when a large amount of new information on remediation is yet to be gleaned. Such programmes have an important function to perform in crystallising questions about sequences of development and methods of teaching. However, for both theoretical and practical reasons, programmes, at this stage in the development of research, need to be seen as preliminary formulations. Practitioners need to be acutely aware of their shortcomings and of the precise scope of their applicability if they are to use them appropriately with their clients. Finally, the whole idea of remediation programmes in terms of the desirability of trying to teach through these means will be questioned.

The Foundations of Programming

Two sets of influences can be seen to operate in the development of language remediation programmes. The first set of influences came from behavioural work with mentally handicapped individuals, in some cases autistic mentally handicapped. These studies accumulated from around 1960 onwards and are reviewed by Garcia and De Haven (1974) and Harris (1975). The studies reflected the general notion that the teaching of language skills is possible, that it begins by teaching the individual to attend, to imitate motor and then verbal responses, to label verbally and finally to build linguistic structures.

Several groups of studies are still influential. The imitation studies showed that it was possible to teach very severely mentally handicapped to imitate noval responses: but they failed to show that teaching motor imitation always transferred to verbal imitative ability (e.g. Garcia, Baer and Firestone, 1971). Nonetheless the belief that this can be done has slipped into clinical practice (Harris, 1975). Other studies showed that mentally handicapped individuals could learn to use generative grammar when imitation training techniques were used. A series of studies by Guess, Baer and their colleagues showed acquisition of plural morphemes, adjectival inflections, verb inflections and other classes (see Harris, 1975, for a review). These studies have been followed by others which have explored methods of training the correct use of syntax by the severely mentally handicapped (Striefel, Wetherby and Karlan, 1978; Wetherby, 1978). The studies represent a valuable resource in programme development.

The second source of ideas and guidance concerning programme development are studies on the language development of children, in particular normal children. Opinions differ somewhat on the necessity for considering such data and on ways in which it might be employed in developing remedial programmes. Some authors, like Miller and Yoder (1972), suggest that normal language development must be *the* basis for remediation. Others emphasise normal development as providing the sequence of goals to be achieved in language development but are happy to use methods based on processes, like imitation-based learning, which are not a crucial means of learning in normal development (Bricker, 1972). Others reject the use of data from studies of normal development of language and pay attention to the analysis of the final products, that is sentences (Carrier, 1974, 1976, 1979; Carrier and Peak, 1975). In practice the majority opinion comes down on using normal development as an overall guide whilst recognising that normative sequences are a product of individuals interacting with their environmental context and not an unfolding biological phenomenon (Kiernan, 1981). Consequently, sequences may be modified to heighten the 'logic' of programme development (Gray and Ryan, 1973; Kent, 1974).

The greatest problem presented by data on normal language development is that it is continually being modified and updated. Since the 1960s it is probably fair to say that the textbooks have needed rewriting on at least three occasions. I will not try to review this material in detail here since it is covered in the first part of this text and in several others (e.g. McLean and Snyder-McLean, 1978). From our point of view what is crucial is the successive recognition of three particular aspects of language development during the 1960s and 1970s and their implications for programming.

Prior to the emergence of Chomsky's work (Chomsky, 1957) and the development of psycholinguistics, the study of early language development was disastrously neglected. Quite often studies were confined to vocabulary counts, with emerging vocabulary classified in terms of parts of speech. The first phase of the modern study of language emphasised the importance of syntactic development, largely as a consequence of Chomsky's work. The second phase, dating from the beginning of the 1970s, represents what has been called the 'semantic revolution'. Broadly speaking it was realised that emerging language could not be understood without analysis of the meanings which the child was trying to express. In practical terms this means that programme planners needed to switch attention from teaching syntactic structures to teaching children how to express propositions about the world which reflected their accumulating knowledge. The initial focus of language training switches away from productive speech to teaching the child how the world works in terms of critical properties and relationships. The focus becomes a focus on understanding, not simply comprehension of spoken language, but understanding of the world *and* comprehension of language, with the level of cognitive development being prior.

The third phase of development of theory involved the opening up of ideas on the functions of language, particuarly social functions, the branch of linguistics called pragmatics (see McLean and Snyder-McLean, this volume). Workers like Bruner (1974) and Bates (1976) developed the notion that spoken language emerges from close inter-personal interaction in which there is a great deal of nonverbal communication. Spoken language builds on early nonvocal communication and subsequently mediates and regulates interactions. Through speech the child can regulate the activities of others in the service of his or her needs and regulate the attention of others through discussion of past, current and future events.

This view of language development is potentially crucial for language programming in arguing that the reason, or at least one of the prime reasons, why children learn language is in order to communicate to others, thereby regulating behaviour (Bates and McWhinney, 1979). The implications of this view for teaching are clear. Teaching should begin from settings in which the child wants to influence the behaviour of others. Teaching should feed the child language structures which can be used to facilitate the child's influence over others and should move to more complex linguistic structures through creating situations in which the child needs to use the structures in order to prevent mis-communication. In other words language remediation should be based around the child's needs to communicate and remedial programmes should emphasise the creation of settings in which these needs are created.

The three views of language development are in most ways complementary and 'disagreements' rest primarily in terms of emphasis. Almost certainly few people would argue with the idea that, in order to communicate, children needs to have the idea that they can influence other people who are around to interact with them (pragmatics), that they have something to say, which expresses needs or knowledge (semantics), and that they have a way of communicating (syntactical skills). In terms of sophistication children can almost certainly communicate when they have simply the idea that they can communicate and that there is someone to respond to their simple needs, even if they have no real syntactic knowledge, that is when they are using one-word,|sign or symbol utterances. More sophisticated children will know different ways of winning and regulating attention, will want to discuss the past, present and future, and will therefore need greater syntactic skills. What emerges clearly is the need to recognise all the aspects of language development in any comprehensive language remediation programme.

However, a word of caution. The account just outlined is grossly incomplete even on our current knowledge of normal development (cf. Yoder and Calculator, 1981) We can not confidently state that there is anything like enough knowledge about normal language development from which to develop complete guidelines. In particular relatively little is known about the language development of handicapped children, especially mentally handicapped children, and consequently there is little on which to base confident applications of findings from the normal child research.

Criteria for Evaluting Language Programmes

In the previous section I described several bases for remedial language programmes for the severely handicapped. The general conclusion which can be drawn is that there is a great deal of information on which to base such programmes but that much of the information is either inconclusive, as in the case of verbal imitation training techniques, or is developing, as in the case of studies of normal language acquisition. This situation obviously creates problems for developers of language programmes. They have to try to establish programmes which reflect well-researched techniques, although these are still being actively evolved. Similarly, for those programme developers who opt for the alternative of basing their programmes on normal language acquisition data, the task of producing viable programmes is difficult given continuously emerging new research.

These are crucial considerations to which I will return. For the moment suffice it to say that practitioners and researchers have felt it worth their while to develop programmes in spite of these difficulties. There are in fact a large number of schemes for language training. In 1975 Fristoe reported on 200 programmes and more have been devised since then.

Several authors have commented on the need to apply standards of evaluation to these programmes which would parallel those required for test standardisation but Fristoe (1975) found that many of the programmes were unsupported by any adequate outcome research. In other terms clinicians were using untested language programmes.

Connell, Spradlin and McReynolds (1977), in commenting on this situation, suggest that programme developers are neglecting their responsibility to provide adequate evidence on the effectiveness of their programmes and that, in using such programmes, clinicians are not meeting 'their obligation to (use) techniques and procedures that have been adequately tested' (1977, p. 564). They suggest that these failures are serious enough to violate codes of professional ethics. The argument may appear to be extreme but it is worth considering. In being subjected to a language programme the handicapped person is being given a 'treatment' analagous in many ways to drug treatment. If it works then the benefits can be substantial, if it is not appropriate then considerable harm can be wrought. Within limits we would not consider using a drug which had not been adequately tested and which did not do what is said it would do, and without adverse side-effects. What is more, the responsibility for providing this crucial information on effects lies with the person producing the drug, in our case, by analogy, the programme developer.

Connell and his colleagues suggest four criteria which programmers should meet before a programme can be accepted as usable. Their criteria are to provide a precise description of all clients used in gathering the data bearing on the programme, thereby allowing the user to know whom the programme can help; to present the percentage of clients who completed each step in the programme, including a description of those who dropped out; information on the mean or median trials to criterion, and the variance of performance on each programme step; and an experimental analysis of the generalisation of trained language behaviours. Muma (1978) criticised the Connell criteria on the grounds that others were more important. He suggested that psychometric criteria fail to assess factors such as the development of deep structure, communicative intent and ecological validity. He argued that descriptive procedures covering the use of acquired communication skills are more important.

In practice this suggests that *both* types of information are of value and that programme developers should at least attempt to provide such evidence if they are to advocate strict use of their programmes. In addition, programmes might be evaluated in terms of the extent to which the methods which they advocate are well supported by research and their methods and sequences accord with developmental considerations, if this is what they aim to do. In the case of programmes which reject the developmental model a clear indication of their rationale and justification for their stance in terms of outcomes would be needed. The ultimate criterion of a good programme is its utility: is it used to good effect by practitioners? Utility depends on a variety of factors including cost, acceptability of format and theory, and ease of use. As we will see utility does not necessarily relate to our other criteria.

We can then come down to a series of questions.

(1) Does the programme say clearly what it can do and for whom?
(2) Does it provide a clear guide to what the user should do?

(3) Does it provide evidence that it will do what it says it will do?
(4) Is its theoretical basis clear and appropriate? In other words if it claims to be based in developmental theory is it up to date and appropriate?
(5) Are the methods advocated optimal in terms of relevant research and theory?
(6) Is it as good as or better than other programmes which aim to achieve parallel goals?

These questions will not be answered in detail but will be used as a background framework for the evaluation of four selected programmes.

Four Programmes

It would clearly be beyond the scope of a chapter of this sort to review all available language programmes for the severely mentally handicapped. McLean and Snyder-McLean (1978) provide a comprehensive review of published programmes, although they are mainly North American. This section will concentrate on representative programmes which are important for different reasons, the consideration of which brings out different points of interest. Two of the programmes are commonly used in the UK and two are likely to be used more in the USA.

The Non SLIP

The first of our programmes originated from a service research context in the USA. It represents just about the tightest programme when evaluated within the criteria suggested by Connell and his associates, who in fact represent the same 'stable'. The Non-Speech Language Initiation Programme (Non SLIP) was developed from the work of Premack and published by Carrier and Peak in 1975. The programme has as its objective the development of language, defined as the appropriate use of linguistic rules through the use of a symbol system. The programme consists of an equipment set and a manual which describes the programme in minute detail. Other publications provide additional outcome information (Carrier, 1976, 1979; Carrier and Hollis, 1979).

Carrier and Peak reject the idea that a developmental approach to language remediation is necessary. They argue that it is more sensible to begin from linguistic analyses of mature syntactic speech. Consequently they select a 'core' sentence, from which they claim all other sentence forms can be derived. They do not quote any support for their selection of the particular core structure used which takes the form of a seven-word sentence of the type 'the boy is sitting under the tree' (first article, first noun, auxiliary, verbing, preposition, second article, second noun). The programme proceeds through a large number of stages, each one of which is outlined in meticulous detail in the manual and in a comprehensive set of work cards. In fact one problem with the programme is that users may feel that it is too restrictive and that it stifles individual originality, a point which the authors address and reject on the grounds that variations are less effective.

One outstanding feature of the programme is that expected completion time, expected percentage errors and times and percentage errors at which performance should be re-evaluated are given for each step. These data are based on the original training group which is described as being severely or profoundly retarded with Adaptive Behaviour Levels at Level IV, with a few at Level III, and Measured Intelligence Levels at Levels IV or V (Heber, 1959). Students ranged in age from 9 to 16 years old and all were institutionalised. 'Some' children are said to have had single words at the beginning of training but none to use more than single-word utterances. Some children suffered mild to moderate problems of co-ordination. Subsequent reports from Carrier have covered children in the same basic population and there is only a little information on the use of the programme with less able children or with children from community settings (Carrier, 1976, 1979; Carrier and Hollis, 1979; Hand and Carmichael, 1979).

The major problem with the Non SLIP programme is that, although steps within the programme are described in substantial detail and certainly meet the Connell criteria, the programme completely fails to suggest how the skills acquired can be generalised. This applies even to the generalisation from the core sentence to other sentences, for example to questions. The programme collapses completely on the Muma criteria, to such a degree that it seems likely that Carrier and Peak would argue that other programmes cover these criteria. However, the problems Muma raises stand especially if Carrier and Peak cannot comment on them. The Non SLIP manual fails to demonstrate that the skills acquired can be generalised and consist of anything more than a simple set of behaviours learned in a non-communicative setting and without functional utility.

In terms of language skills the programme concentrates entirely on syntax. The programme addresses itself only to the teaching of a single social function of language, how to answer questions, and that function only in a single restricted setting. The originators of Non SLIP do not pay direct attention to the possibility that the student may not 'realise', or may have to learn that language can be used to satisfy needs, ask questions, draw attention, etc. In other words the crucial question of communicative use is ignored.

In terms of finance the programme package is costly. In addition teachers and other users may be put off by the high degree of programme structure. Surveys of use of nonvocal systems suggest that the programme may be used only rarely (Goodman, Wilson and Bornstein, 1978; Kiernan, Reid and Jones, 1982).

The Non SLIP programme is probably the best documented programme in the area of language remediation. Nothing else even approaches its sophistication. The fact that the programme fails to meet several crucial criteria serves, as much as anything else, to illustrate some of the problems of adequate programme construction, but as it stands it is really only a limited syntax programme rather than a general language programme. In summary, Non SLIP excels in clearly stating whom it is for and what it can do. It provides painstakingly clear guidance on what the user should do, and evidence that the programme will do what it is supposed to do. The theoretical basis of Non SLIP is clear, although the rationale behind the choice of core sentence is not clear. In terms of teaching method the programme embodies much behavioural research. Where it falls down is in not showing how responses can be generalised. In practice this means that students are taught only one sentence type and one social function of language, that is answering questions. No comparative data are presented to indicate whether the programme is more or less effective than others.

The Makaton Vocabulary

This language programme had its origins in the development of British Sign Language (BSL) for use with mentally handicapped adults in subnormality hospitals (Cornforth, Johnston and Walker, 1974; Cornforth and Woods, 1972). Initially the vocabulary was a straightforward core of useful signs but the Revised Makaton Vocabulary (Walker, 1976a) is presented as a language programme. The structure of the programme is determined by the sequence of groups of items known as Stages, and associated teaching methods are described in a manual (Walker, 1976a, b).

The importance of the Makaton Vocabulary lies in its widespread use in the UK. Beginning in 1976 Walker and her colleagues have run a large number of workshops for practitioners on the Vocabulary. Walker

(1978) estimated that, by that time, 1,000 people had attended workshops. BSL signs within the Makaton Vocabulary are used by the overwhelming majority of schools for the severely mentally handicapped (Reid, Jones and Kiernan, 1983). Jones, Reid and Kiernan (1982) found that, in 1980, 51.5 per cent of schools for the severely mentally handicapped used the Vocabulary in a strict way, 41.5 per cent used it flexibly and the remainder used it in different ways depending on the child's needs. Comparable data were provided by schools for the physically handicapped. These data suggest that the Makaton Vocabulary is being used on a widespread basis as a language programme.

At its simplest level the Revised Vocabulary consists of a list of around 350 words. Other materials provide pictures of the corresponding signs (Walker, 1976a, 1977). The list is arranged in nine Stages each comprising around 40 words. Clearly, users could employ the list in two ways. They could use it as a 'sign bank', ignoring the order of Stages. This approach is not accepted by Walker (1978), who states that the 'need to adhere to the stages of the Vocabulary is *vital*' (1978, p. 178, Walker's italics) in order that the language programme is preserved. Although Walker and Armfield (1981) soften this position somewhat the pressure is still against deviation from the Stage sequence. The purposes of the Vocabulary are given by Walker (1978, p. 178). She sees it as providing a basic vocabulary for communication and language learning which follows normal development, is appropriate for mentally handicapped people, and can be combined into short phrases thus providing a basic and useful communication system.

The Language Programmes are divided into two groups. Walker (1976b, p. 7) talks in terms of 'high dependency' mentally handicapped individuals for whom special programmes are suggested. These programmes involve only the first two Stages of the Vocabulary. The full Makaton Vocabulary is seen as suitable for those 'mentally handicapped individuals above the level described above for whom it is hoped that sign language will provide a means of communication' (Walker, 1976b, p. 7). The term 'high dependency' is commonly applied to individuals who are either severely physically handicapped and mentally handicapped or who show substantial behaviour problems along with mental handicap. No further clarification of criteria for inclusion in the two types of programme is provided here or elsewhere.

The content of the nine stages is described by Walker (1978). This analysis will concentrate on the first two Stages of the Vocabulary since it is these Stages which are said to apply to the more handicapped. In addition concentration on these Stages highlights several of the crucial features of the Vocabulary. A more general critique is offered by Byler (1983).

Vocabulary selection in the 1973 version of the Vocabulary was based on a combination of factors, including experience of the workers who developed the programme and on vocabulary studies by Mein and O'Connor (1960). The study had been done in the late 1950s by recording ten-minute conversations between adult mentally handicapped men in subnormality hospitals and one of the experimenters. After three or four interviews conversation ran out and pictures, used initially in a study of the vocabulary of normal five year olds, were used as stimulus material. This material was used on the apparent assumption that, since Mental Age was comparable, interests would be comparable.

Mein and O'Connor constructed a Core Vocabulary of 218 words. The overlap of the Core Vocabulary with the Revised Makaton Vocabulary is, however, limited. Only 39.7 per cent of Makaton Vocabulary words are in the Core Vocabulary and some of the core words which were not might have been of use (e.g. all, back, by, curtain, floor, far, pea, pick, round, seeing, wall). No reasons for exclusion are given. Secondly, there is no clear relationship between the mean percentage use of words according to Mein and O'Connor and the placement of words in the Makaton Vocabulary. It would be expected that more frequently used words would be included in the earlier stages, but in fact the average percentage use for the first five stages are all in the mid 70 per cents. Less commonly used words are included in Stages 6 and 7 but not in Stage 8.

Since 1976 several vocabularies have been produced which bear on the Makaton selection, including Fristoe and Lloyd's (1980) lexicon based explicitly on developmental work with normal children by Holland (1975) and by Lahey and Bloom (1977). Fristoe and Lloyd group their items into relational signs which are not object specific, like 'all-gone', 'more', 'this/that/those', and signs that relate to many objects such as 'play', 'stand' and 'heavy'. Their third group is of substantive signs including proper nouns, pronouns and nouns as names of objects. The vocabulary is also organised in terms of semantic categories.

Fristoe and Lloyd, in common with Walker, place relatively less emphasis on substantives as part of their vocabulary. These are seen as more child and situation specific and consequently as substitutable, a suggestion which Walker also makes but which is often ignored by therapists who adhere closely to the Vocabulary. Relational terms in the Fristoe-Lloyd vocabulary are, as noted, derived explicitly from work on normal development.

In terms of the semantic categories derived from the Fristoe-Lloyd vocabulary the Makaton stages considered here do not cover 'recurrence of objects and actions' (more) or 'noting existence' (this, that, those), although 'here' and 'there' are included. Other items in the Fristoe and Lloyd relational list which do not appear in the Makaton list include several terms for actions or objects (bring, get, help, kiss, make, open, play, throw), actions involved in locating objects or self (fall, put, run, walk, up, down) and attributes (big, broken, happy, heavy, open). Many of these differences are arguably unimportant, reflecting minor preferences. The proportion of relational to substantive words is more worrying, given the Makaton claim for developmental viability. Around 35 per cent of Makaton items are relational (allowing for multiple meanings) as opposed to around 48 per cent of Fristoe-Lloyd items.

Of greater concern is the absence of *clear* coverage of several semantic categories described by Fristoe and Lloyd. It is generally accepted that children express various categories of negation. These constitute rejection, expression of nonexistence or disappearance ('all gone', or 'no . . . '), cessation of action ('no' as in 'stop' or 'finish') and prohibition of action ('no'). The Makaton Vocabulary includes 'no' as an item in Stage 1. However, neither the Vocabulary itself nor the Stage 1 Language Programme (Walker, 1976b) acknowledges these multiple meanings. The Language Programme refers to the use of 'yes' and 'no' but in no way indicates their precise meaning (1976b, p. 1-2). What emerges here is a failure to relate the Makaton Vocabulary to research on language development, in this case semantic development, despite its claim to be so based. It will be seen that this problem recurs later.

The Language Programmes at each Stage are highly variable in the detail which is provided. In most cases 'programmes' comprise lists of suggested activities, like taking walks, constructing story books or colouring pictures (Stage 3). This sometimes reduces to a level where suggestions are minimal. For example, in teaching the adjectives 'clean' and 'dirty' the suggestion is that they should be taught 'when practical opportunities occur, e.g. patients clothes or hands are dirty sign "hands dirty – go and wash" ' (Walker,1976, p. 2-2). Or, in teaching the words 'We (us) they (them)' Walker suggests that the signs should be used 'as they occur appropriately. No specific work required. Patients will use them as and when they are ready' (1976b, p. 4-3). The same considerations apply to other words, for example 'sorry' and 'now'.

Teaching programmes are included in Stage 1 and in several later Stages. For example, specific programmes are included to teach colour and prepositions. The standard method of teaching employs pictures of objects, or miniatures where appropriate. Typically the method consists in teaching students to answer questions. Bailey (1978) has argued that this static method is counter-developmental. Certainly as it stands the method emphasises teaching individuals to answer questions about pictures and little else is programmed explicitly.

Some omissions from suggested programmes are peculiar given that we are talking about language programmes. There are no suggestions at all concerning methods of teaching linguistic rules. In fact this area is only mentioned in passing, e.g. 'encourage signing in phrases. Provide plenty of examples yourself for them to learn from' (1976b, p. 5-2).

As noted the 'High Dependency' mentally handicapped are dealt with separately in a two-page section of the Language Programmes. The section introduces the idea of teaching signs for objects and suggests that this be followed by teaching signed instructions, social responses and signs for people. She also suggests that for 'this level of patient only Stages 1 and 2 and some nouns, that is food from Stage 3 would be relevant' (1976b, p. 10-2). This excludes the teaching of 'more'.

From the viewpoint of teaching method the Walker programmes are in general fairly vague. As we have seen the only clearly described method is a question-and-answer technique which she refers to on several occasions in the programmes and which has become the hallmark of Makaton teaching. In one form or another pictures or objects are shown, students are asked to name them and prompted and rewarded as necessary. Beyond this form of teaching Walker encourages users to respond to 'spontaneous' signing. This term clearly refers to all of the other functions of language. However, just as we saw in the case of semantic relations, the programme fails to reflect developmental research relevant to the analysis of social function. As in the case of the Non SLIP programme Makaton runs into serious problems in recommending teaching within a very restricted framework. The danger with the approach is that, unless the student already has varied concepts of the social functions of language, the programme may lead only to skills in answering questions in set situations.

The Language Programmes as published do not contain data on rates of learning or expected outcomes. The only data which have been published by Walker and her associates relate to studies completed in the early 1970s concerning the initial introduction of sign language with deaf mentally handicapped adults living in subnormality hospitals. Cornforth, Johnston and Walker (1974) provide gross outcome data from studies in four hospitals. Walker (1973, 1977) provides further data on the group from one of these hospitals (see also Bicknell, 1974). A survey of use by Walker (1978) and data from a survey of use and outcome (Kiernan, Reid and Jones, 1982) completes the list of published data. The data from the early studies illustrate the rapid acquisition of BSL signs by deaf mentally handicapped adults. Many of these students were relatively able (cf. Bailey, 1978) and in the Walker study which covers one of the groups in detail, students were able to identify up to 110 of the 145 signs used prior to teaching (Walker, 1973). These data do not bear on the Makaton Vocabulary as a language programme.

Walker (1978) suggests that the system can be used with 'subjects having mental ages as low as 18 months'. She suggests that these students are able to learn the first two or three stages, but presents no data to back this claim. She also suggests that a child or adult with a mental age of 2-2½ years will understand and sign 'most of Stages 1 to 4 in three months' and in six months will 'know them thoroughly'. No supporting evidence is quoted. Walker's claims are widely at variance with the data reported by Kiernan, Reid and Jones (1982), who found that, amongst ESN(S) Day School children in programmes lasting from 6 to 18 months, the median child could understand between 11 and 20 signs and use between 5 and 10. Even when more competent children (speaking children) were involved, the number of signs understood was only between 21 and 30 signs and they used between 11 and 20. Stages 1 to 4 include around 150 signs. On the available data Walker's estimates seem to be exaggerated.

It is now possible to answer the series of questions in respect of the Makaton Vocabulary. The programme does indicate in broad terms the range of subjects covered, but it is not clear exactly what it is designed to do. The Language Programmes give only general guidance on procedures and no data are provided on the effectiveness of the Language Programmes. The Makaton Vocabulary claims to be developmentally based but pays scant attention to work on semantic relations or social function and says nothing about the teaching of syntactic skills. As has already been noted, descriptions of methods are in general vague and the one method described in full relates to only a narrow social function, answering questions. No comparative data on outcome are presented by the proponents of the programme. Data from a survey of use of systems by Kiernan, Reid and Jones (1982) showed no clear differences attributable to the way of using the Vocabulary, that is with strict use of Stages or flexible use.

Given these conclusions some comment must be offered in explanation of the popularity of the Vocabulary in UK schools. Four factors seem to be important. Firstly the Vocabulary is linked with the successful introduction of signing and, for many practitioners, the illustrations of Makaton Vocabulary signs is their only guide to sign form (Walker, 1977). Success resulting from the use of BSL signs can easily be confounded with success resulting from use of the Vocabulary. Secondly the Vocabulary is 'user friendly'. It is learned readily in one-day workshops and presented in a single sheet of paper with associated illustrations. The Language Programmes are brief and undemanding. Thirdly, substantial claims are made for the Vocabulary. Walker and Armfield (1981) see it as 'a complete language programme' which 'provides a guide for even the most experienced language development teacher or therapist as well as those new to vocabulary development' in terms of 'graded stages [which] permit communication to begin immediately at the most basic level' (1981, p. 20). Finally, the use of the Vocabulary is supported in schools and clinics by regional representatives, part of whose function is apparently to ensure that the Stage structure is followed.

The proponents of Makaton Vocabulary have made a substantial contribution in introducing signing to a large number of special schools. However, the Makaton Vocabulary and associated Language Programmes do not seem to be defensible when assessed as a language programme.

Functional Speech and Language Training for the Severely Handicapped.

In 1976 Guess, Sailor and Baer produced a language programme based in part on their research of the early 1970s. The pack comprises four work-books with associated scoring and summary forms. The programme is outlined by Guess, Sailor, Keogh and Baer (1976). It involves two 'tracks', a Preacademic track for severely handicapped children who could benefit from an academically orientated programme and a Community Living track for students who need basic social and survival communication skills. The Preacademic track covers content areas such as possession, colour, size, relations and morphological grammar (plurals, suffixes, tenses and inflections); the Community Living track covers social skills, self-help and conversational skills.

The programme is organised along five 'dimensions' — which are functional aspects of speech and language. Guess and his colleagues first of all address the reference function of language. The next three dimensions refer to social aspects, the control function of language ('I want thing or action' or 'I want action with thing'), self-extended control (the student asking for further information) and integration (related to information seeking and dialogue). The final dimension is Reception, understanding of language, which Sailor and his colleagues see as in many ways secondary to productive language training. The programme is laid out in substantial detail with each training step outlined in terms of the specific language to be used and expected. Sample outcomes are described and criteria for successful completion are indicated.

The Guess, Sailor and Baer programme is impressive in terms of its clear presentation. It is also impressive in that it represents one of the few well-developed programmes which emphasise the social function of language. This emphasis arises from its behaviouristic origin rather than from any influence from linguistics (see Blackman, this volume). However, as McLean and Snyder-McLean (1978) point out, the social functions taught within the programme are very limited. The programme fails to emphasise the use of language in the regulation of social interaction and co-operation.

One of the problems with the programme relates to a central difficulty with all formalised programmes. Guess, Sailor and Baer share with Carrier and Peak (1975) the assumption that language can best be taught in formalised settings with generalisation to informal settings. Generalisation has always been a problem with language programmes (cf. Harris, 1975). There are several possible reasons, one of which is that workers often expect generalisation across social functions, for example from answering questions to drawing attention to needs. An alternative approach is suggested from the work on social function in language development, in which programming would begin from meaningful social contexts. The difficulty is that these contexts will be defined by individual needs and interests and so will be difficult to codify in terms of formal programmes.

The problem is highlighted by Sailor (1982) in an analysis of the reasons for failure of students on the Guess, Sailor and Baer programme. He reports that around 40 per cent of the population failed to acquire the initial vocabulary. Sailor argues that the reasons lay in the overemphasis on formal stimulus control techniques and a consequent de-emphasis on inherent motivational factors. In other words that the students did not learn to communicate because they were not motivated to do so. Sailor emphasises the need to provide the child with functional competence through language as motivation to learn.

In terms of our questions the Guess, Sailor and Baer programme fares better than the other two which we have examined. The programme is clear in its aims and procedures, although unclear on whom it will be useful with. Some evidence that it will do what it says it will do is available, although not in the programme pack itself (Warren, Rogers-Warren, Baer and Guess, 1980; Sailor, 1982). Much of the evidence on effectiveness is indirect, deriving from the studies on acquisition of generative grammar mentioned earlier. Theoretical bases are clear but can be criticised on the grounds of being narrow. In addition to not covering pragmatic analysis the authors set aside specific consideration of the relationships of language to cognitive development (McLean and Snyder-McLean, 1978). This may well account for some of the problems described by Sailor since users have no guide to the level of cognitive development which the student should have if the programme is to be of value.

The Derbyshire Language Scheme

This scheme has been developed from classroom practice in the UK by Knowles and Masidlover (1982). It was first publicised in the mid-1970s and has been revised several times. Currently, the scheme is a combined system of language assessment and remediation which bases itself on the language skills of normal children but which emphasises that normal development should be seen as a 'flexible framework'.

The scheme begins from a Rapid Screening Test and an extensive assessment of comprehension skills (the Detailed Test of Comprehension) which starts with assessing responses to single questions (e.g. 'give me the spoon') and goes up to the understanding of complex questions, past and present verb forms and prepositions. Assessment is designed to be completed by the person using the scheme partly because assessment is seen as a means of sensitising the practitioner to the dimensions of the scheme and partly to check the assessment procedure. In practice it is necessary to check the procedure since, apparently, neither reliability nor validity of the tests of comprehension have been established. On the basis of the assessment pupils are assigned to one of three stages, the Early Vocabulary or Single Word Level, the Simple Sentence Stage, or the Grammar and Complex Sentence Stage. Together these constitute ten levels for teaching.

The approach to teaching is characterised in three ways. Firstly it is activity-based. The two manuals consist in large part of descriptions of suggested activities related to levels and teaching groups. The emphasis is on communication within game-like situations rather than on formal teaching. Secondly the emphasis is on teaching comprehension skills within these settings. In essence the teacher is, initially, urged to ensure that the child knows the relationships of objects and people within the teaching setting. This is then very much a semantically-based approach.

The third feature of the approach is that the teaching of expressive skills is effected through role reversal. Once the child is thought to know how to 'play the game' the teacher or therapist takes a passive role and the student is encouraged to play the role of teacher. This strategy deals effectively with the type of problem which has been identified in previous programmes where the social function of language which is taught is very restricted. Here the child learns to regulate the speech and general behaviour of others as well as assuming the passive role of answering questions. The authors are quite explicit in the aims of the scheme. They say that it 'aims at facilitating the "use" of language to control other people, obtain objects and to obtain information' (1982, p.13). They exclude the use of language in self-regulation, recall of the personal past or planning for the distant future from coverage in the programme.

The level of specificity in describing teaching procedures is very variable. Some are fairly specific, describing apparatus, layout of programme and interactions, although in no case is the level of specificity as detailed as that seen in the Non SLIP or Guess, Sailor and Baer programmes. The majority are fairly non-specific and rely mainly on suggestions embedded in examples. None of the activities have associated data illustrating their effectiveness. The Derbyshire Language Scheme is embodied in large loose-leaf volumes and a spiral bound assessment text. It is introduced in a workshop which normally lasts for three days. Supplementary material is provided for participants to either complement or replace sections of the Manuals.

In terms of the questions identified the Derbyshire Scheme fares, on balance, as well as the other programmes looked at. It does say quite clearly what it is for. The device of using an assessment prior to teaching serves both as a means of placing students and a way of introducing the main themes of the scheme. The aims of the programme are outlined. The approach to structuring teacher activity avoids specificity. Like the Makaton Programmes activities are suggested rather than components being described in detail. However, the Derbyshire Scheme provides many more activities and in greater detail than does the Makaton Programme. Nonetheless a great deal is left to the teacher in terms of filling out most activities.

The Derbyshire Scheme, like most others, does not provide any evidence that it will do what it says it will do. The user is asked to accept activities as having been evolved in practice to a level where they are potentially useful. There are no data comparing the approach with others. The theoretical bases of the scheme are not made explicit in the manuals. Nonetheless the approach is impressive in the way it accords with deductions from a semantic theoretical approach and the way in which it copes with the problem of giving language a social function, albeit one which is somewhat restricted. The take up of the Derbyshire Scheme in terms of teacher and therapist interest appears to be high. The materials are 'user friendly' in being easy to read and in suggesting activities rather than prescribing them.

Discussion

Several conclusions seem to follow from this review. It has been argued that there are data which can be used as foundations for remedial language teaching. These data come from experimental studies and from data on normal child development. Additionally, theoretical formulations from behavioural work and from psycholinguistics can be utilised. It has been noted that workers within the behavioural tradition often reject the use of developmental models. However, it needs to be recognised that rejecting of the theoretical model does not imply denial of the existence of behaviour described by that model. The Guess, Sailor and Baer programme is explicity behaviourally based but does a good job of covering the type of behaviour seen as central by pragmatically oriented linguists.

The programmes analysed vary in the degree to which they draw on available sources. Of the two developmentally oriented programmes the Makaton Vocabulary fails to meet criteria of credibility in developmental terms. It has been suggested that it does not reflect key considerations embedded in semantic theory or work on the social function of language and it simply ignores programming of syntactic development. Its developmental base lies only in a broad correspondence of initial vocabulary, defined only in terms of lexical items and not meaning, and in a broad correspondence to normal cognitive development, referred to as language concept, embodied in the overall stage sequence. The Derbyshire Scheme fares far better in terms of reflecting developmental theory. It has been seen that although apparently semantic in its theoretical basis, it copes with at least some of the questions raised from considering the social function.

Of the four programmes considered only one, the Non SLIP programme, succeeds in meeting the criteria developed by Connell and his colleagues (Connell, Spradlin and McReynolds, 1977). Even the relatively tight Guess programme is only now being evaluated. Similarly none of the programmes have been evaluated for their relative value against others. Two of the programmes are vague about whom they are going to be effective with. Sailor's paper (Sailor, 1982) shows the consequence of this in his report that 40 per cent of students failed to get established in the programme. In the case of the Non SLIP programme it is arguable that the kind of criteria provided by Carrier and Peak, in terms of general functioning levels, may be irrelevant. Data on the ability to participate in and relate to the question-answering function of language may be more crucial. The whole question of cognitive prerequisites is raised by this and the Guess programme.

There are fascinating possibilities raised by this kind of discussion. One lies in the diametrically opposed approaches of Guess, in emphasising production, and Knowles and Masidlover in emphasising comprehension. Presently, there is insufficient evidence to evaluate the relative value of these differing attacks. Another is the neglected area of user-acceptability and related dimensions.

The discussion of programmes leads inevitably to the question of whether it is actually possible to formulate an adequate programme. Developers appear to be caught on the horns of a dilemma. Do they adopt a theoretical and methodological base and then try to gather honest data to test the viability of their system? If they do this they will take so long to develop their programmes that the theoretical and methodological bases will almost certainly be out of date when they produce their final packages. Alternatively they could publish, and be damned on the grounds that they have no evidence to support the specific recommendations which they are offering. This approach is justifiable only if the stance is made clear. The analogy with new drugs needs to be taken seriously and practitioners warned that programmes need to be treated as sources of possible ideas rather than prescriptions.

Two methods of escape from the dilemma should be considered. The first would be to produce 'programmes' as loose structures of ideas, subject to continuous modification and evaluation in light of new work and experience. This approach may be feasible so long as the initial framework remains compatible with new ideas and so long as there are personnel to service the developing scheme. In relation to the first point it is arguable that some of the basic orientations in some behavioural work, as represented for instance by the Carrier programme, are incompatible with more recent work on the social function of language. This programme represents the child as an essentially passive learner, not as an active initiator, and in fact should be seen as relating only to the initiation of the use of syntactic rules.

The problem of personnel is much more difficult and leads us to an alternative approach to changing teacher and therapist behaviour. In essence language remediation programmes are devices through which the crystallised knowledge of one individual or group of individuals is transmitted to others. It has been suggested that there are substantial and inherent problems in producing language programmes which are up-to-date and well researched. At any given stage programmes are provisional formulations and most programme developers do not have the time, resources or application to meet the need for continuous revision. Given this situation the alternative to trying to produce programmes is to enhance the general level of flow of new information to practitioners through general in-service training. Clearly such training needs to be structured so as to prevent a chaos of minor applications of transient ideas. But in essence the development of language remediation programmes is an attempt to restructure the thinking and behaviour of practitioners which is arguably bound to fail. The alternative to trying to provide pre-digested solutions is progressively to raise the overall level of practice thorugh the continuous flow of informed discussion and ideas.

References

Bailey, R.D. (1978) Makaton success: fact and artefact, *Apex, 6*, 18-19

Bates, E. (1976) *Language and Context*, Academic Press, New York

——and McWhinney, B. (1979) A functionalist approach to the acquisition of grammar, in E. Ochs and B.B. Schiefflin (eds.), *Developmental Pragmatics*, Academic Press, New York

Bicknell, D.J. (1974) Communication with the deaf mentally handicapped in hospital, *Proceedings of the Royal Society of Medicine, 67*, 1029-31

Bricker, W.A. (1972) A systematic approach to language training, in R.L. Schieflbusch (ed.), *Language of the Mentally Retarded*, University Park Press, Baltimore

Bruner, J.S. (1974) From communication to language – a psychological perspective, *Cognition, 3*, 25-287

Byler, J.K. (1983) The Makaton Vocabulary: An analysis based on recent research, submitted for publication

Carrier, J.K. (1974) Nonspeech noun usage training with severely and profoundly retarded children, *Journal of Speech and Hearing Research, 17*, 510-17

——(1976) Application of a nonspeech language system with the severely handicapped, in L. Lloyd (ed.), *Communication Assessment and Intervention Strategies*, University Park Press, Baltimore

——(1979) Application of functional analysis and a nonspeech response mode to teaching language, in R.L. Shiefelbusch and J.H. Hollis (eds.), *Language Inter-*

vention from Ape to Child, University Park Press, Baltimore
———and Hollis, J.H. (1979) Recent research on the Non-speech Language
Initiation Program (non-SLIP), in R.L. Schiefelbusch and J.H. Hollis (eds.),
Language Intervention from Ape to Child, University Park Press, Baltimore
———and Peak, T. (1975) *Non-Speech Language Initiation Program*, H & H
Enterprises, Lawrence, Kansas
Chomsky, N. (1957) *Syntactic Structures*, Mouton, The Hague
Connell, P.J., Spradlin, J.E. and McReynolds, L.V. (1977) Some suggested criteria
for evaluation of language programs, *Journal of Speech and Hearing Disorders*,
42, 563-7
Cornforth, A.R.T., Johnston, K. and Walker, M. (1974) Teaching sign language to
the deaf mentally handicapped, *Apex, 2,* 23-5
———and Woods, M.M. (1972) Subnormal and deaf, *Nursing Times*, 10 February
Fristoe, M. (1975) *Language Intervention Systems for the Retarded. A Catalogue
of Original Structure Language Programmes in Use in the United States*,
State of Alabama Department of Education, Montgomery
———and Lloyd, L.L. (1980) Planning an initial expressive sign lexicon for
persons with severe communication impairment, *Journal of Speech and Hearing
Disorders, 45*, 170-80
Garcia, E., Baer, D.M. and Firestone, I. (1971) The development of generalised
imitation within topographically determined boundaries, *Journal of Applied
Behaviour Analysis, 4*, 101-13
———and De Haven, E.D. (1974) Use of operant techniques in the establishment
and generalisation of language: a review and analysis, *American Journal of
Mental Deficiency, 79*, 169-78
Goodman, L., Wilson, P.S. and Bornstein, H. (1978) Results of a national survey
of sign language programmes in special education, *Mental Retardation, 16*,
104-6
Gray, B. B. and Ryan, B. A. (1973) *A Language Programme for the Non-Language
Child*, Research Press, Champaign, Illinois
Guess, D., Sailor, W. and Baer, D.M. (1976) *Functional Speech and Language
Training for the Severely Handicapped (Parts 1-4)*, H and H Enterprises,
Lawrence, Kansas
———Sailor, W., Keogh, W. and Baer, D.M. (1976) Language development
programs for severely handicapped children, In N. Haring and L. Brown (eds.),
Teaching the Severely Handicapped — a Yearly Publication (Vol II), Grune
Stratton, New York
Hand, V. and Carmichael, W.T. (1979) Teaching a symbol system to nonverbal
severely retarded children, unpublished Advanced Diploma dissertation,
University of London Institute of Education
Harris, S.L. (1975) Teaching language to non-verbal children — with emphasis on
problems of generalisation, *Psychological Bulletin, 82*, 565-80
Heber, R. (1959) A manual of terminology and classification in mental retarda-
tion, *American Journal of Mental Deficiency Monograph Supplement*, No. 64
Holland, A. (1975) Language therapy for children: some thoughts on context and
content, *Journal of Speech and Hearing Disorders, 40*, 514-23
Jones, L.M. Reid, B.D. and Kiernan, C.C. (1982) Signs and symbols: the 1980
survey, in M. Peter and R. Barnes (eds.), *Signs, Symbols and Schools: An Intro-
duction to the Use of Nonvocal Communication Systems and Sign Language in
Schools*, National Council for Special Education, Stratford
Kent, L.R. (1974) *Language Acquisition Program for the Retarded or Multiply
Handicapped*, Research Press, Champaign, Illinois
Kiernan, C.C. (1981) Behaviour modification and the development of communi-
cation, in P. Mittler (ed.), *Frontiers of Knowledge in Mental Retardation, Vol.*

1. Social, Educational and Behavioural Aspects, University Park Press, Baltimore
——Reid, B.D. and Jones, L.M. (1982) *Signs and Symbols: A Review of Literature and Survey of Use of Non Vocal Communication Systems*, University of London Institute of Education Studies in Education, No. 11, Heinemann, London
Knowles, W. and Masidlover, M. (1982) *Derbyshire Language Scheme*, private publication, Ripley, Derbyshire
Lahey, M. and Bloom, L. (1977) Planning a first lexicon: which words to teach first, *Journal of Speech and Hearing Disorders, 42*, 340-59
McLean, J.E. and Snyder-McLean, L.K. (1978) *A Transactional Approach to Early Language Training*, Charles E. Merrill, Columbus, Ohio
Mein, R. and O'Connor, N. (1960) A study of the oral vocabularies of severely subnormal patients, *Journal of Mental Deficiency Research, 4*, 130-43
Miller, J. and Yoder, E.D. (1972) On developing the context for a language teaching programme, *Mental Retardation, 10*, 9-12
Muma, J. (1978) Connell, Spradlin and McReynolds: Right but wrong! *Journal of Speech and Hearing Disorders, 43*, 549-52
Reid, B.D., Jones, L.M. and Kiernan, C.C. (1983) Signs and symbols: the 1982 survey of use, *Special Education: Forward Trends, 10*, 27-8
Sailor, W. (1982) Functional competence: issues in the teaching of a first vocabulary to severely handicapped students, paper presented to the 6th International Conference of the IASSMD, Toronto
Striefel, S., Wetherby, B. and Karlan, G.R. (1978) Developing generalised instruction following behaviour in severely retarded people, in C. Meyrs (ed.), *Quality of Life in Severely and Profoundly Mentally Retarded People in Research Foundations for Improvement*, American Association on Mental Deficiency, Washington, DC
Walker, M. (1973) An experimental evaluation of the success of a system of communication for the deaf mentally handicapped, unpublished Master's Thesis, University of London
——(1976a) *The Makaton Vocabulary, (Revised Edition)*, Royal Association in aid of Deaf and Dumb, London
——(1976b) *Language Programmes for use with the Revised Makaton Vocabulary*, private publication, Chertsey, Surrey
——(1977) Teaching sign language to deaf mentally hadicapped, in *Language and the Mentally Handicapped 3*, BIMH, Kidderminster
——(1978) The Makaton Vocabulary, in T. Tebbs (ed.), *Ways and Means*, Globe Educational, Basingstoke
——and Armfield, A. (1981) What is the Makaton Vocabulary? *Special Education, 8*, 19-20. Also in M. Peter and R. Barnes (eds.), *Signs, Symbols and Schools*, National Council for Special Education, Stratford
Warren, S.F., Rogers-Warren, A., Baer, D.M. and Guess, D. (1980) Assessment and facilitation of language generalisation, in W. Sailor, B. Wilcox and L. Brown (eds.), *Methods of Instruction for Severely Handicapped Students*, Paul H. Brookes, Baltimore
Wetherby, B. (1978) Miniature languages and the functional analysis of verbal behaviour, in R. Schiefelbusch (ed.), *Bases of Language Intervention*, University Park Press, Baltimore
Yoder, D.E. and Calculator, S. (1981) Some perspectives on intervention strategies for persons with developmental disorders, *Journal of Autism and Developmental Disabilities, 11*, 107-23

PARENTS AS THERAPISTS: A CRITICAL
REVIEW

Patricia Howlin

Involving parents in the treatment of their children is by no means a novel concept. In the period following the Second World War, when personnel shortages were marked, Munro (1952) and Davis (1947) both used group training procedures to teach parents better child management techniques, and Williams (1959) describes one of the earliest behavioural studies in which parents carried out a simple but effective programme to extinguish severe bedtime crying in a two-year-old. The 1960s saw a rapid proliferation in the use of parents as 'change agents' for their own children (Johnson and Katz, 1973) and parents steadily became involved in a wide range of programmes designed to reduce maladaptive psychotic, and neurotic behaviours. (For reviews of studies in this area, see Berkovitz and Graziano, 1972; O'Dell, 1974; Yule, 1975; Gath, 1979.)

The apparent success of parent training in the elimination of behavioural disturbance was followed by the involvement of parents in programmes designed to increase children's developmental skills, particularly in the areas of language and communication. Amongst the earliest studies utilising parents as language therapists are those of Welsh (1966), Hawkins, Peterson, Schweid and Bijou (1966), Gardner, Pearson, Bercovici and Bricker (1968) and Johnson and Brown (1969). Since these early studies parents have been extensively involved in language training programmes.

The Role of Parents in Therapy

The advantages of employing parents as therapists for their own children are manifold. Firstly, such an approach is highly economical and allows a one-to-one mode of therapeutic intervention, which, at least in theory, can be continued throughout the child's waking day, and which would be unavailable in many other settings (Hemsley, Howlin, Berger, Hersov, Holbrook, Rutter and Yule, 1978).

Secondly, it avoids problems of generalisation and maintenance

197

which are particular pitfalls in any programme with handicapped children. Many children with learning difficulties show very little generalisation from one setting to another, nor do gains necessarily endure once treatment ceases. Lovaas, Koegel, Simmons and Stevens (1973), for example, showed that despite the marked improvements in language made by autistic children in a highly-staffed clinic setting, these gains were lost rapidly when the children returned home. Only if parents were actively involved in treatment throughout, were newly learned language skills transferred to the home setting.

Thirdly, parents, because of their unique involvement with the child, are likely to be highly motivated to persist and succeed in treatment. They are likely, also, to have control over far more powerful reinforcement contingencies than any outside therapist (Tharp and Wetzel, 1969).

Finally, and perhaps most importantly, it is postulated that changing the child's verbal environment is crucial for the success of language training procedures. Thus, by definition, parents or principal caretakers must be involved in treatment if it is to be effective.

The Effects of Parents' Speech to Children

The Language Environment of Normal Children: the Search for Causal Relationships

The verbal environment to which normal children are exposed has been investigated in many studies (Farwell, 1973; Vorster, 1975; Snow, 1977; Snow and Ferguson, 1977; Howe, 1981), and it is clear that the way in which adults talk to children is strikingly different to adult conversation. As well as differences in tone and prosodic emphasis there is a greater use of didactic utterances, repetitions, interrogatives, imperatives and expansions (Brown, 1973; Cross, 1977; Newport, Gleitman and Gleitman, 1977; Rutter, 1980). The high frequency, and apparently universal nature, of these features in adults' talk to young children have led to the assumption that such linguistic markers may be specifically designed to facilitate children's language acquisition (Moerk, 1972; Snow and Ferguson, 1977).

Observational studies have found a number of associations between maternal speech and language development in children. Thus, the use of questions, extensions and expansions of the child's speech tends to be positively correlated with language acquisition (Furrow, Nelson and Benedict, 1979; Olsen-Fulero, 1982; Barnes, Gutfreund, Sattersly and Wells, 1983). A frequent use of imperatives and negation by parents, on the other hand, is associated with inhibited development (Clarke-Stewart, 1973; Nelson, 1973; Newport *et al.*, 1977; Kaye and Charney, 1981). However, the assumption that a causal relationship exists between maternal speech and children's language development is unwarranted on a number of grounds. Firstly, simple correlational studies, such as those cited above, do not demonstrate causality, merely associations. Secondly, the 'universality' of the findings is questionable because of the very small and socially homogeneous samples of mother-child pairs investigated, (i.e. usually white, middle class and well educated). Thirdly, the development of mother-child interaction studies, the ways in which speech samples are collected and the limited number of parameters used to analyse interaction also raise many problems (Barnes, *et al.*, 1983).

Experimental studies have generally failed to demonstrate convincing links between mother's speech and children's subsequent language development. Thus, Brown and Hanlon (1970) found that increases in the amount of verbal reinforcement used by mothers had apparently little effect on language learning. Cazden (1965) and Feldman (1970) found similar negative results when expansions of children's utterances were deliberately increased. And, although Routh (1969), Hursh and Sherman (1973), Nelson (1977), and Garcia and Wallace (1977) all found that specific changes in the style of adult utterances could selectively increase verbalisations or syntax acquisition in young children, the linguistic structures acquired were very limited in both range and number. Shatz (1982) concludes that there is very little evidence of any direct causal links between linguistic input and subsequent language development. Moreover, a number of studies indicate that individual differences in children's styles of discourse or level of comprehension may well influence adult speech rather than vice versa (Lieven, 1978; Van Kleek and Carpenter, 1980; Nelson, 1981). Barnes *et al.* (1983) suggest a compromise solution; namely that although what is learned is strongly determined by the characteristics of the learner, certain features of the input are better suited to the optimal development of these characteristics than others. This would seem to be the wisest interpretation of the available data, although, again, there is no supporting experimental evidence as yet.

The Language Environment of Linguistically Handicapped Children

Despite the failure to demonstrate causality between language input and language development in normal children, a number of studies of linguistically delayed children suggest that inadequacies of parental speech may be holding back language development (Kogan and Tyler, 1973; Marshall, Hegrenes and Goldstein, 1973; Buium, Rynders and Turnure, 1974). However, much of this apparent 'deviance', in maternal speech tends to disappear if normal and handicapped groups are adequately matched (Rondal, 1978). Cunningham, Reuler, Blackwell and Deck (1981) found that mean length of mothers' utterances (MLU) is directly related to children's mental age, and several other studies, too, have failed to find MLU differences if children are matched for mental or language age (Frank, Allen, Stein and Meyers, 1976; Rondal, 1978; Wolchick and Harris, 1982). Moreover, even for children brought up in very 'deviant' linguistic environments — as in the case of hearing children with deaf parents — only minimal exposure to a normal language environment is necessary to ensure that language develops appropriately. This, too, suggests that the fact of having a poor parental model can hardly be the explanation for seriously delayed language learning (Schiff, 1979).

Nevertheless, although the length or frequency of parental utterances to retarded children does not seem to be restricted in any way, the results of a number of studies indicate that 'normal' styles of interaction may be less efficient in eliciting or encouraging language from retarded children (Cunningham *et al.*, 1981; Lazky and Klopp, 1982; Peterson and Sherrod, 1982). Thus, although parents cannot be held responsible in any way for the delayed development of their children, it is possible that modifying their interactions with their children might help to create a more beneficial language environment. Hence, their direct involvement in language intervention programmes would seem to be important for success.

The Involvement of Parents in Language Therapy

The Techniques Used

Although a number of language programmes involving parents have made use of modelling procedures, rather than emphasising reinforcement techniques (e.g. Seitz and co-workers, 1974, 1976), direct operant training procedures have proved by far the most popular of techniques. The effectiveness of these methods in hospital settings was first described by Lovaas (1966) and Sloane and MacAulay (1966), and shortly afterwards similar techniques began to be employed in the home. To begin with, interventions tended to focus predominantly on the extinction of inappropriate utterances or the use of reinforcement to increase appropriate vocalisations or imitative speech (Gardner *et al.*,

1968; Johnson and Brown, 1969; Goldstein and Lanyon, 1971; Mathis, 1971; Nordquist and Wahler, 1973). Subsequent studies have tended to be far more sophisticated, involving individual assessment of children's language deficits and specific teaching of psycholinguistic rules. In addition they have frequently made use of carefully designed play activities and a general restructuring of the adult-child interaction to facilitate a language-learning environment at home (Jeffree and Cashdan, 1971; Jeffree, Wheldall and Mittler, 1973; MacDonald, Blott, Gordon, Spiegel and Hartmann, 1974; Cheseldine and McConkey, 1979; Howlin, 1980a; Harris, Wolchik and Weiss, 1981; Jones, Clements, Evans, Osborne and Upton, 1983).

Recently, too, there have been successful programmes to teach non-verbal forms of communication to children who have not responded to vocal training (Salvin, Routh, Foster and Lovejoy, 1977; Casey, 1978). All the studies discussed in this review have made use, to some extent, of basic behavioural techniques such as reinforcement, prompting and shaping procedures and, in certain cases, punishment to extinguish inappropriate speech. In most instances the techniques used have been individually tailored to suit the needs and skills of the particular children involved in treatment, although in some of the group studies training in behavioural techniques has, of necessity, been more genera-lised. (For a discussion of the basic techniques used see Harris, 1975; Yule and Berger, 1975; Howlin, 1980b; Harris and Wolchick, 1982.)

The Children Involved

The range of children involved in language programmes at home is con-siderable. Amongst children receiving help have been those with articu-lation disorders (Carrier, 1970; Shelton, Johnson, Ruscello and Arndt, 1978), hearing problems (Bennett, 1973; Carpenter and Augustine, 1973; Seitz and Marcus, 1976), language delays (Whitehurst, Novak and Zorn, 1972; Miller and Sloane, 1976; Stevenson, Bax and Stevenson, 1982; Lombardino and Magnan, 1983), elective mutism (Nolan and Pence, 1970), behavioural disturbances (Russo, 1964; Welsh, 1966; Johnson and Brown, 1969; Seitz and Hoekenger, 1974), and mental re-tardation (Jeffree, Wheldall and Mittler, 1973; Salzburg and Villani, 1983; McDonald *et al.*, 1974; Cheseldine and McConkey, 1979; Sandler, Coren and Thurman, 1983). Autistic children, too, have received considerable attention, because of the widespread language difficulties amongst this group and the importance of language devel-opment for prognosis (see Harris *et al.*, 1981; Howlin, 1981a; Koegel, Rincover and Egel, 1982, for reviews). In addition, there have been a

number of studies which have involved parents in more general programmes to help their handicapped children. These have not necessarily
assessed linguistic improvements separately, although the training of
language skills has been an important goal for parents (Bidder, Bryant
and Gray, 1975; Revill and Blunden, 1979; Callias, 1980; Sandow,
Clarke, Cox and Stewart, 1981).

There are also many reports of programmes for children whose impoverished language skills are the result of poor environmental conditions. The majority of 'Head Start', 'Follow Through' or associated
home-intervention programmes have assessed language progress in conjunction with other developmental changes, although intervention
procedures have generally been designed to improve the child's overall
level of functioning rather than focusing on specific language disabilities. These studies encompass a very wide group of children and the
methods of intervention used are also varied. Since they do not, on the
whole, involve children with developmental language delays but deal
rather with problems resulting from poverty and inadequate stimulation, they will not be covered in the present chapter. Details of these
studies, however, can be found in the following reviews: Gray and
Wandersman 1980; Palmer and Anderson, 1980; Zigler and Valentine,
1980; Rhine, 1981.

Levels of Parental Involvement

Although there is now general agreement that parents should, wherever
possible, be involved in the treatment of their own children, the extent
of this involvement remains variable. At the simplest level parents may
merely be 'encouraged' to carry out the recommended techniques,
whilst most of the direct therapy is carried out by professionals in the
clinic or child's school. For example, in the Nolan and Pence study
(1970) of an electively mute child, parents had access to the child at
weekends only. Similarly, in the studies by Gardner *et al.* (1968), Salvin
et al. (1977), Bloch, Gersten and Kornblum (1980) with autistic
children and Seitz and Hoekenger (1974) with disturbed and retarded
children, parents played a very minor role in treatment and their own
efficiency as therapists was not assessed.

In a number of other reports parents have taken a more active role in
treatment but, again, all training and assessment was carried out in the
school or clinic rather than at home. Examples of this type of approach
are the studies of Welsh (1966), Johnson and Brown (1969), McConkey, Jeffree and Hewson (1979), Lombardino and Magnan (1983) with
retarded and developmentally delayed children, and those of Goldstein

and Lanyon (1971) with autistic children.

In another group of studies, training and assessment have taken place initially in a clinic or school setting, but then — either because of the failure of treatment effects to generalise to the home, or because a gradual shift to the home had been planned from the outset — further intervention and some observational measures have been completed at home. Amongst studies combining a home and clinic-based approach, are those by Carrier (1970) and Raver, Cooke and Apolloni (1978) with articulation problems; MacDonald *et al.* (1974) and Salzburg and Villani (1983) with Down's Syndrome children; and work with autistic children by Wolf and colleagues (1964, 1967), Kozloff (1973), Lovaas *et al.* (1973), Nordquist and Wahler (1973), Casey (1978) and Koegel, Glahn and Nieminen (1978).

Because of the necessity, reported in many studies, to transfer treatment to the home in order to ensure continuation of progress, recent intervention programmes have tended to concentrate almost entirely on home-based treatment and assessment. Again, even in some home-based programmes much of the treatment has been the responsibility of professional therapists with parents playing a subsidiary role (Stevenson *et al.*, 1982). In contrast, in the studies by Jeffree and Cashdan (1971), Bennett (1973), Whitehurst *et al.* (1972), Miller and Sloane (1976), Kaufman and Kozloff (1977) and Hemsley *et al.* (1978) members of the child's own family have taken on responsibility as the major therapists. Bennett (1973), for example, successfully used the 4-year-old sister of a deaf girl as therapist.

The extent of parents' autonomy in implementing programmes is also variable. In the Whitehurst *et al.* (1972) and Miller and Sloane (1976) studies, parents were given very specific advice about the use of prompting and reinforcement techniques. Clements and his colleagues (1980, 1982), Jeffree and Cashdan (1971), Kaufman and Kozloff (1977) and Hemsley *et al.* (1978) gave parents broader programmes to follow, as well as providing them with a general grounding in behavioural techniques. In the latter study the parents were encouraged to modify existing programmes and to design new ones as appropriate. They were responsible, too, for much of the data gathering.

Contact with therapists in all these studies was maintained at regular intervals during treatment, but since frequent home visits by therapists are not always possible other studies have reported positive results with much less professional involvement. Thus in Mathis' (1971) report of an autistic boy, the child was never seen by professional workers at all. His mother attended the clinic for advice about treatment whilst carrying out training and data collection unaided at home. This appeared to be highly successful, although a similar approach used by Carpenter and Augustine (1973), indicates that the totally unsupervised collection of data by parents tends to produce more favourable results than standardised follow-up assessments would seem to warrant.

One way of avoiding this problem, yet at the same time reducing the amount of professional involvement required, is the use of group training, where discussion of treatment and the assessment of results is carried out during group sessions in the clinic, whilst parents carry out treatment unaided at home. Amongst studies of language training involving parental groups are those of Harris *et al.* (1981) with autistic children, and Mash and Terdal (1973), Sandler *et al.* (1983) with mentally retarded and developmentally delayed children.

It is clear that many different levels of parental training and involvement are subsumed under the title of 'parent training programmes'. In some studies, in fact, parental training and responsibility is virtually nil, with parents simply playing the role of onlookers or rather low-level technicians. In others, parents have played a much more vital role. Indeed one study, amongst those cited, was completed and written entirely by the child's father (Park, 1974).

The Evaluation of Language Training Studies

The sheer numbers of language modification studies which have appeared in the recent literature and the range of language disorders which have been treated by parents, using predominantly behavioural techniques, would seem to be testimony to the efficacy of such treatment methods. However, because of the inadequate experimental design of many of the studies, their effectiveness is less well established than might be assumed. It is important to bear in mind that the majority of the studies discussed are, essentially, single case reports. Admittedly, they are almost all highly successful but few journals willingly publish unsuccessful case studies.

Experimental Design in Small Group or Single Case Studies

In any treatment study, for behavioural control to be adequately demonstrated, certain basic requirements must be met. Amongst these are baseline measures of problem behaviours, detailed descriptions (allowing replication of the study) of therapeutic techniques, reliable and objective assessments of behavioural change and the use of control groups or, in the case of single case studies, systematic variation of treatment contingencies (see Eysenck, 1961; Sherman and Baer, 1968; Gardner, 1969; Pawlicki, 1970; Berkowitz and Graziano, 1972; Kazdin, 1973a; McDonagh and McNamara, 1973; Risley and Baer, 1973). Whilst reliable data reporting and adequate descriptions of treatment are obvious requirements in any therapeutic study, the inclusion of suitable experimental controls is particularly important in studies of language modification. This is because language delay is a developmental problem and is likely to improve with time, even if therapy is not available. Thus, whether or not the changes observed following treatment are any greater than might be expected by chance is frequently difficult to ascertain. Good baseline measures are obviously important but simply demonstrating improvements in pre- and post-treatment assessments is not sufficient, in itself, to demonstrate the effectiveness of therapy. The most reliable method of ascertaining the efficacy of any intervention is to match experimental subjects with untreated, matched controls. However, adequately designed control studies are time-consuming, expensive, and may require more personnel than are normally available in a clinic setting. In addition, individual case studies to assess the feasibility of new treatment procedures are often required before large-scale group studies can be carried out. The implementation of reversal or multiple baseline designs with single case studies reduces the need for control groups but even these procedures may present problems. Reversal techniques, which involve a return to baseline conditions after treatment contingencies have been in force for some time, may be difficult to apply because parents are often reluctant to give up an apparently effective procedure. Moreover, for some children, the ability to use language rapidly becomes reinforcing in itself, and once language skills become well established the removal of extrinsic reinforcers may have little effect. Multiple baseline designs, in which specific behaviours are modified selectively or in a predetermined sequence offer an alternative approach, but are based in the assumption that the behaviours selected for systematic treatment are functionally independent — an assumption which is not always valid (Kazdin, 1973b; Yule, 1974).

Nevertheless, despite the problems involved, unless basic experimental requirements are fulfilled, the effectiveness of treatment cannot be established. Thus, even if full-scale reversal or multiple baseline techniques are difficult to implement, modified procedures, such as partial reversal or 'multiple probes', as suggested by Horner and Baer (1978), are required.

To assess fully the success of intervention follow-up measures, too, are required. There is little value in a treatment programme if improvements are lost immediately it is discontinued. Finally, since language modification has been attempted with a very heterogeneous group of children, details of individual characteristics, such as age, IQ and diagnostic criteria are required in order to determine which children respond best to treatment (Garcia and De Haven, 1974; Yule and Berger, 1975).

The Assessment of Studies Involving Parents as Therapists

In a previous review of language modification, involving both clinic and home-based intervention, Howlin (1979) found that of 167 studies reported between 1964 and 1978 involving autistic, mentally retarded and other linguistically handicapped groups, very few actually met the basic experimental criteria detailed above. Most did provide adequate details of treatment and gave some limited information about the children involved, such as age, sex and diagnosis (although even this information was inadequate in about 10 per cent of studies and details of IQ levels were given in only 30 per cent). Eighty-seven per cent provided adequate baseline data, and 73 per cent reported their findings in an objective form (i.e. by graphs or tables). However, only 38 per cent had assessed the reliability of their observations or recording measures; only 53 per cent applied any form of experimental manipulation or used untreated controls, and only 24 per cent provided follow-up data.

The present review includes studies of language training, with parents as therapists, which have been reported or cited in major journals of language and behaviour therapy between the years of 1964 (when such studies were first reported) and the time of writing (1983). Table 9.1 presents details of these studies, according to the level of experimental sophistication employed.

Single Case Reports

Of almost 50 studies reviewed, the first group of nine are simply general descriptions of the types of methods used. No baseline data are available nor are the results of individual programmes reported in any detail, although Clements *et al.* (1980) give information about a single case study; Rose (1974) reports on the number of assignments completed by parents following group sessions, and Attwood (1977b) gives figures for rates of attendance at group workshops.

A further five studies describe the effects of treatment in individual cases but baseline information are inadequate or lacking entirely and the reports of progress are mainly anecdotal. Goldstein and Lanyon (1971) and Seitz and Marcus (1976) attempt some objective data presentation but omit any reliability figures. The Nolan and Pence (1970) study compared the progress of an autistic boy during behavioural treatment to his lack of previous progress whilst receiving psychotherapy, but as this information is retrospective and anecdotal it can be given little weight.

In the next group of five studies, which provide some baseline data, that of Lombardino and Magnan (1983) produces information only on parental measures, not on children's speech. The remaining four do make use of graphs or tables to present their data but only Seitz and Hoekenger (1974) provide reliability data. McConkey *et al.* (1979) describe two cases in which multiple baselines were used but no such manipulations were employed in the assessment of the other eight children in the study.

Follow-up information in all these studies, as in the first group of descriptive reports, is mainly lacking or is entirely anecdotal; Salvin *et al.* (1977) are the only authors to record the actual numbers of words and signs maintained at follow-up.

The next group, of 13 studies in all, is generally more sophisticated. All provide baseline information, objective data recording and, in every case except one, have assessed the reliability of their measures or used previously standardised assessments. All employ some type of experimental manipulation although the sophistication of the techniques employed is variable.

The Use of Multiple Baselines or Experimental Probes

Mathis (1971) assessed verbal progress in an autistic child in both trained and untrained conditions but although data are presented in graph form the reliability of the measures — which were gathered entirely by the mother — is not assessed. Bennett (1973), too, tested generalisation to untrained probe items but did not then go on to train these specifically which would have demonstrated more powerful experimental control. Harris *et al.* (1981) used a short (3-9 week) assessment period to monitor verbal changes in autistic children prior to and following the onset of treatment. No gains were observed during the assessment-only condition, whereas improvements occurred rapidly once treatment commenced.

Other studies have made use of multiple baseline techniques —

Table 9.1: An Evaluation of Language Therapy Programmes at Home

	Diagnosis	N	Age	IQ	Baseline	Objective data	Reliability data	FU	Notes
A. Descriptive only: No data									
1969									
Terdal *et al.* (a & b)	Retarded behaviour Disorder	?	?	?	—	—	—	—	
1971									
Schopler & Reichler	Autistic	?	?	?	—	—	—	—	
Hislop	?	?	?	?	—	—	—	—	
Leverstein	?	?	?	?	—	—	—	—	
1976									
Rose	Retarded	33	?	?	—	—	—	—	
1977									
Attwood (a)	Retarded	25	<5y.	?	—	—	—	—	
(b)	MH & PH	18	Mixed	?	—	—	—	—	
1980									
Clements *et al.*	Retarded	40+	Av. 28m	<78	(Outcome details in later studies)				
B. Single Case Studies: No Baseline									
1966									
Welsh	Delayed language	2	?	?	—	—	—	—	Anecdotal
1970									
Nolan & Pence	Elective mute	1	10y	'Normal'	—	—	—	—	"
1971									
Goldstein & Lanyon	Autistic	1	10y	?	—	Single graph	—	—	"
1976									
Seitz & Marcus	Multiple handicap	1	20m	Retarded	—	Tables	—	—	—

Year	Study	Diagnosis	N	Age	IQ	Anec-dotal				Type of manipulation
1978	Raver et al.	Articulation disorder	1	3.5y	?		—	—	—	No FU but examined generalisation to untrained stimuli
C. Single Case Studies Baseline data										
1969	Johnson & Brown	Slow development	1	1.9y	60-70	+	+	—	Anecdotal	
1974	Seitz & Hoekenger	Retarded and/or disturbed	4	2-4y	?	+	+	+	—	
1978	Salvin et al.	Autistic	1	5y	63	+	+	—	?	
1979	McConkey et al.	ESN(s)	10	Av = 53m	Av = 53	+	+	—	—	Multiple baseline in 2/10 children
1983	Lombardino & Magnan	Developmental delays	6	1-4y	?	On parents only	+	+	—	
D. Single Case Studies + Experimental Manipulation										*Type of manipulation*
1964/1967	Wolf et al.	Autistic	1	6-9	?	⊦	+	+	Anecdotal	Reversal
1968	Gardner et al.	Autistic	1	6y	?	+	+	+	"	Multiple baseline
1971	Mathis	Autistic	1	8y	?	+	+	+	+	Multiple baseline
1972	Whitehurst et al.	Delayed	1	3	117	+	+	+	Anecdotal	Reversal

	Diagnosis	N	Age	IQ	Baseline	Objective data	Reliability data	FU	Type of manipulation
1973									
Bennet	Deaf	1	3y	?	+	+	+	Anecdotal	Generalisation to probe items
Carpenter & Augustine	Deaf	1	22m	?	+	+	+	"	Multiple baseline
	Speech delay	1	8y	Normal					
Kozloff	Austic	4	mxd	?	+	+	+	+	Multiple baseline
Nordquist & Wahler	Autistic	1	4	?	+	+	+	+	Reversal
1976									
Miller & Sloane	Nonverbal	3	6-12	?	+	+	+	Single assessment	Multiple baseline & generalisation to unsettings
1978									
Casey	Autistic	4	6-7	?	+	+	+	+	Multiple baseline across subects
1981									
Harris *et al.*	Autistic	11	Av. 49m	Av. 30	+	+	+	Anecdotal	Pre-treatment Assessment period
1983									
Salzburg & Villani	Down's	2	3½	50	+	+	+		Multiple baseline
Sandler *et al.*	Mixed	21E	Av. 45m	?	?	?	?		Brief report only. No details of children's speech

									Notes
E. Control Group Studies									
1970									
Carrier	Articulation problems	10E 10C	4-7	?	?	?	?	?	Brief report only
1971									
Jeffree & Cashdan	ESN(s)	15E	11y	<50	+	+	+	—	
1973									

Year / Author	Population	Sample	Age	IQ					Notes
1973									
Mash & Terdal	Retarded	45E 5C	4-10y	50-55	+	+	+	−	Comparative data only on mothers', not children's speech
Jeffree *et al.*	Down's	1E 1C	4y	?	+	+	+	1 assessment	
Lovaas *et al.*	Autistic	20	mxd	?	+	+	+	+	
1974									
McDonald *et al.*	Down's	3E 3C	<5	?	+	+	+	+	
1977									
Brasel & Quigly	Deaf	36E 36C	10-18	?	+	+	+	−	cf. between manual and verbal training
Kaufman & Kozloff	Autistic	7E 4C	?	?	+	+	+	1 assessment	
1978									
Shelton *et al.*	Articulation problems								
Hemsley *et al.*	Autistic	16E 30C	3-11	60+	+	+	+	+	see also Howlin (1981) FU by Holmes *et al.* (1982)
1979									
Cheseldine & McConkey	Down's	7	Av. 62m	?	+	+	+	−	
Cooper *et al.*	Language delay	E₁ 50 E₂ 69 C₁ 39 C₂ 20	2y-10½	?	?	+/−	−	−	Multiple baseline + later controls
1980									
Bloch *et al.*	Autistic	12E 14C	3-4y	<50	+	+	+	?	−
1982									
Clements *et al.*	Mentally retarded	14E 17C	<5 >5	72 45	+	+	+	−	see also Jones *et al.* (1983)

1982

	Diagnosis	N	Age	IQ	Baseline	Objective data	Reliability data	FU	Notes
Clements *et al.*	Preschool	14E	5	72	+	+	+	−	See also Jones *et al.*
	Mentally retarded	17C	5	45					
Stevenson *et al.*	Delayed	11E	2½-3½	80-90	+	+	+	−	
		11C							
Koegel *et al.*	Autistic	?	2y.10m	$\bar{x}$ MA 2.7y	+	+	+	+	

1983

Jones *et al*   (continuation of Clements *et al.*'s report)

Notation:

+ = Adequate information
− = No information
? = Results not adequately reported

selectively training one aspect of language behaviour at a time (Gardner *et al.*, 1968; Carpenter and Augustine, 1973; Kozloff, 1973); one subject at a time (Casey, 1978), or working in one experimental setting at a time (Miller and Sloane, 1976; Salzburg and Villani, 1983). All these studies appear to demonstrate the effectiveness of the experimental procedures employed in selectively changing language skills. However, as they generally utilise a variety of techniques – including reinforcement, prompting and modelling and often specific language programmes, too, the particular components of treatment which are important for success remain unclear.

Cheseldine and McConkey (1979) employed a rather different intervention design. To begin with, they gave parents a language objective to work towards with their children but provided no instructions as to how they might attain this goal. All parents spontaneously altered their language strategies and three were very successful in achieving the goals set. Two of the unsuccessful parents were then taught specific training strategies and their child made greater progress in imitation and spontaneous use of words than the remaining two parents, who continued as before. This study suggests that for some parents, at least, it may not be training in the use of prompts and reinforcements which affects the progress of their child. Instead, simply being given guidance on which aspects of language development they should try to modify may be sufficient to bring about improvements.

Reversal Techniques

Only a minority of studies have attempted to apply reversal procedures. Whitehurst *et al.* (1972) combined reversal and multiple baseline techniques in a study of a three-year-old child with delayed language. A high level of prompting and general conversation by the mother resulted in rapid improvements in the child's speech. Other conditions, such as low-level prompting but high conversation or vice versa, were less successful, whilst a return to baseline conditions of infrequent prompts and little conversation resulted in a marked drop in the rate of acquisition of new words by the child. The child's verbal behaviours did not, however, regress to the initial baseline level, when he was observed to use only one word and a variety of grunts. This study indicates that reversal procedures can be used to demonstrate effective experimental control without actually causing the child to lose new skills entirely. In fact, Hamblin, Buckholdt, Ferritor, Kozloff and Blackwell (1971) present data which suggest that after a brief reversal period the rate of learning may be more rapid than prior to reversal. Nordquist and

Wahler (1973) applied a combination of multiple baseline and reversal procedures. Reversal periods were kept very brief (usually only a few sessions) but indicated clearly the effectiveness of experimental techniques. Wolf, Risley and Mees (1964) also used reversal techniques in their work with an autistic boy. In this study, however, the recording and experimental manipulation were carried out in the clinic setting, rather than at home by the parents.

Unfortunately, in all these studies attention has been directed principally to changes observed during the experimental period only and follow-up information, if provided at all, is mainly anecdotal. Although Miller and Sloane (1976) did include a single follow-up assessment, this measured the frequency of parental prompts, not the child's responses. Harris *et al.* (1981), in an otherwise well controlled study, did not carry out a formal follow-up, athough the authors do suggest that no further improvements were made once treatment ceased.

Group Studies

Of the studies using control groups, some have assessed differences between treatments whilst others have examined progress in experimental children and untreated control groups. Carrier (1970), working with children with articulation problems, compared a combination of articulation training and reinforcement by parents with sound imitation training. He concluded that articulation training was significantly more effective but unfortunately no statistics are presented to validate this claim. Brasel and Quigley (1977) compared manual communication training by parents of deaf children with oral communication methods and found that children in the manual group made significantly greater gains in a wide variety of areas. Lovaas *et al.* (1973) and Koegel *et al.* (1982) compared the progress of autistic children, whose parents were involved in treatment, with those whose parents had not received training. The Lovaas study did not set out to assess the two groups separately but in a retrospective analysis of data they concluded that gains were not maintained unless parents had been actively involved. Koegel *et al.* (1982) explored this finding more systematically. They found few differences in immediate, post-treatment measures but at follow-up children in the parent-training group were far more advanced in all areas, including verbal skills, than those in the clinic group, who had actually lost some of the skills acquired during training. Unfortunately, although the graphs presented by the authors are impressive, statistical information about the significance of these differences is not provided. Details of the time intervals between pre- and post-treatment and follow-up assessments are also lacking. Statistical analysis is inadequate, too, in several other studies comparing treated with no-treatment groups (cf. Cooper, Moodley and Reynell, 1979). For example, Bloch *et al.* (1980) report fully on all the changes found in the experimental children, who apparently reached criterion on assessment measures more frequently than controls. However, they discuss only selected changes in the control group. MacDonald *et al.* (1974) report greater gains in the mean utterance length of Down's Syndrome children receiving language training at home than in controls but, again, the control group did show some gains which are not taken into consideration.

Cambell and Stanley (1966) make it clear that calculating differences in pre- and post-test scores for experimental and control groups separately, thereby showing that the gain in the treated group is 'significant' whilst the gain in the untreated group is 'not', is not sufficient to demonstrate that treatment is effective — particularly if both groups make some gains. It is necessary, at the very least, to calculate differences in *gain* scores or, preferably, to use regression or analysis of covariance techniques, which take into account initial differences between groups.

In other studies, in which the progress of families involved in group training is compared with waiting list or untreated controls (Mash and Terdal, 1973; Sandler *et al.* 1983), improvements in mothers' speech to children are reported but since no information is provided about changes in children's speech it is not possible to evaluate the effects of treatment.

In studies where improvements between children have been adequately assessed the effects of treatment are often disappointingly small. Stevenson *et al.* (1982) found that experimental and control groups showed improvements on all the tests used (the Reynell, the EPVT and the Griffiths Scales) but differences in change scores were not significant. The only measure on which the experimental group showed any superiority to controls was the Reynell Expressive Scale, on which four controls showed a decline in standard scores compared with none of the experimental group. Kaufmann and Kozloff (1977) found significant changes in the experimental parents' skills as language therapists but no changes in children's speech were recorded. Jeffree and Cashdan (1971) also failed to find differences in most of the group measures they used. Both experimental and control children showed improvements on the Reynell Language scales, whilst both groups showed a decline in their scores on the Columbia and Peabody

Tests. The only scores showing a differential improvement in the experimental children were on the Renfrew Articulation Test, although no mention of articulation was made to mothers during the period of the programme. Similarly, Clements *et al.* (1982) failed to find any significant differences between experimental and control groups on the Reynell Language Scales. On the Griffiths test, the language scales failed to differentiate between groups, although the experimental group showed significant improvements on the Personal-Social and Eye-Hand Co-ordination Scales. The authors also report that, although language changes were generally non-significant, the improvements which did occur were generally limited to increases in the children's vocabulary. The length and complexity of children's utterances did not change.

Finally, in the study by Hemsley *et al.* (1978), in a study employing a short-term, no-treatment group, and a long-term control group, in which parents were given advice about language training on an out-patient basis but were never seen at home, a number of interesting findings emerged. Following the first six months of treatment, children in the experimental, home treatment group showed significant changes in gain scores, as compared with the controls, on several language measures, including frequency of utterances and their use of communicative speech. Echolalic and stereotyped utterances showed a significant decline. However, although the experimental group showed greater improvements than controls in their level of language competence, as measured by the Reynell tests and their use of various morphemes and transformations, the differences between the groups were generally none significant. When compared with a longer-term control group, at the end of 18 months of treatment, experimental children again performed better on almost every language measure. However, there were few significant group differences in language level and only a limited number of significant differences in their use of communicative speech. There were, however, larger and significant differences between groups on the majority of the *behavioural* problems assessed.

Unlike most of the other control studies cited, this investigation followed up cases and controls two years after the cessation of treatment. Again, it was found that parents in the experimental groups were more successful in dealing with behavioural problems than controls but intervention over language problems did not differ (see Holmes, Hemsley, Rickett and Likierman, 1982).

The Effectiveness of Language Training Procedures

This review of studies of language modification by parents suggests not only that parents can be trained as therapists for their own children, but that essential experimental manipulations can be modified to suit home-based projects as well as those conducted in clinics or special units. However, it is apparent that not all programmes do meet the necessary standards of experimental research. It is also apparent that the success of many programmes tends to be negatively correlated with the levels of experimental sophistication employed.

Thus, almost all the purely descriptive studies conclude with glowing reports of the benefits which their programmes can provide. Those with simple pre-post treatment measures are also highly optimistic, with reports of 'important gains' (Goldstein and Lanyon, 1971), increases in 'positive responding' (Seitz and Marcus, 1976), and even 'normal speech' (Nolan and Pence, 1970). Studies employing multiple baseline or reversal designs are equally optimistic in their views of the effectiveness of therapy, although the language skills involved in these studies tend to be more circumscribed. Thus, there are reports of increases in the numbers of spontaneous words recorded, or in the frequency of imitation, or rate of communicative utterances. Similarly, rates of echolalic or stereotyped speech are recorded as decreasing following systematic correction or extinction programmes.

In contrast, the studies employing control groups produce disappointingly few significant results. Any gains which are reported tend to be associated with behavioural or social development; changes in language are few and, if they do occur, are limited to simple linguistic skills, such as improvements in articulation or vocabulary. More fundamental aspects of language, such as the semantic, syntactical or transformational complexity of utterances, show little significant change (Howlin, 1981a; Clements *et al.*, 1982). And, even if short-term group differences do occur, longer-term follow-ups indicate that many significant treatment effects are short-lived (Hemsley *et al.*, 1978).

Given the disappointing results of control studies, is there, in fact, any evidence that language therapy is effective? Certainly, studies using multiple baselines and reversal techniques do seem to demonstrate that some skills change predictably once language programmes are initiated. In addition, despite the failure to find overall group differences, almost all the studies employing controls report that more experimental than untreated children show improvements. Moreover, losses in language skills, which are occasionally reported for control

children, do not tend to occur in the experimental groups. The conclusion that language training is totally ineffective is difficult to
reconcile with the more positive results of well conducted, single case
studies. It may be that the small sample size of many of the studies cited
may account for some of the failures to find significant differences. The
approach to the analysis of the data, too, may overlook important
changes in *individual* children.

Individual Differences in Response to Treatment

Although group differences between experimental and control children
are disappointingly small, the 'swamping' effects of group data may at
times obscure changes which are occurring, at least in some children.
The importance of taking into account individual differences has only
rarely been considered in the language training literature (Howlin,
1981a; Clements *et al.*, 1982), and perhaps the key question should be,
not whether language training works, but for whom it works. More
systematic assessment of the children involved in language intervention
programmes is badly needed but, despite frequent pleas for better
descriptions of subjects who do *and do not* respond to treatment (Yule
and Berger, 1975), details of the chronological, mental and language
ages of children involved are frequently lacking, or are presented simply
as average scores. Howlin (1981b), for example, found that although
overall group differences were not significant, certain children in the
experimental group, notably those who were at the single-word stage of
development, showed very marked changes in comparison with controls
at a similar level. In contrast, non-speaking children, párticularly those
who had low scores on measures of comprehension, social skills and
play, made very little progress.

The failure of non-speaking children to respond to treatment has
been reported in a number of other studies (cf. Harris *et al.* 1981) and
although it is possible to teach children to use their existing language
skills more effectively, language intervention is unlikely to improve
basic linguistic competence. Koegel *et al.* (1982), for example, found
that although it was relatively easy to train vocalisations based on
phonemes already in the child's repertoire, sounds which were not
present prior to training proved extremely difficult to teach.

Many studies have reported that echolalic children tend to respond
better to intervention that any other group. Lovaas (1977b), for example, states that as a consequence of operant training procedures such

children 'acquired . . . strikingly complex language behaviours'. Howlin (1981a, b) also found that echolalic children seemed to respond best to treatment. However, when echolalic children amongst the control group were assessed at follow-up it was found that they, too, were doing almost as well as children in the experimental group. These results suggest that children who are using some communicative speech, even if this is predominantly echolalic, are likely to make steady gains in language skills, whether or not they are exposed to special treatment. Thus control groups are essential if erroneous conclusions about the effectiveness of treatment are to be avoided.

Outcome Measures

In addition to paying more attention to individual characteristics and their relation to outcome, assessment measures, too, should be sensitive to changes both in the child's speech and other areas of development.

Language is a highly complex skill, covering very many aspects of functioning, and assessment based on only one or two parameters may fail to identify important changes which are occurrring in other areas. A number of studies, for example, note that although language *level* does not change radically (Jeffree and Cashdan, 1971; Howlin, 1981a, b; Clements *et al.*, 1982; Jones *et al.*, 1983), improvements in the frequency of children's utterances, in their vocabulary, and in their articulation, do occur. Such changes may be limited but they may, nevertheless, have a marked effect on the child's ability to communi-cate and may greatly improve social interactions (Hemsley *et al.*, 1978). Even if these improvements are short-lived, so that control groups catch up on such measures after a time, there may be short-term advantages to experimental children in terms of fostering social devel-opment or preventing behavioural disturbance. Thus, as well as increas-ing the range of language measures employed in analysis, extending assessments to other areas of functioning may produce more encoura-ging results. Forehand, Guest and Weil (1979) suggest that, in addition to employing suitable outcome measures, it is important to analyse the *relationships* between these measures, which may well differ across subjects.

The conditions under which language changes should be measured also poses some difficulties. Many studies indicate that children's lingui-stic performance under 'free play' and standardised conditions may vary considerably and that formal assessments may underestimate their true level of competence (Prutting, Gallagher and Mulac, 1975). Obviously, standardised tests are necessary for comparisons across studies or between groups but they may be less sensitive to discrete improvements in language skills and are unlikely to reflect accurately the child's functional use of language in the home setting. A combination of standard tests, together with reliable and objective measures assessing spontaneous language, is more likely to monitor real changes in performance than formal testing alone can do (Cantwell, Howlin and Rutter, 1977; Gerber and Goehl, 1980).

Treatment Effects

If we accept that language training does work, at least with some children, the next question is what particular aspects of the programme are most effective? Almost all the studies described above have employed a combination of training techniques, including reinforcement, modelling, prompting and correction, but which of these is crucial for success is undetermined. Whitehurst *et al.* (1972) suggest that the frequency of prompting by parents is particularly important, though this has not been experimentally validated. Other authors (Howlin, 1981a; Clements *et al.*, 1982) have stressed the importance of following normal developmental sequences in teaching syntactic and semantic rules. Howlin also suggests that teaching should be related to the child's mental age. This seems sensible enough advice, but again there is no hard evidence to suggest that certain sequences of training are better than others. Many of the intervention programmes involve the general restructuring of the child's environment in order to foster language usage, as well as enouraging parents to work towards specific language goals and parents frequently report that being given help in organising and structuring their time with their handicapped child is beneficial in itself (Hemsley *et al.*, 1978; Clements *et al.*, 1982; Holmes *et al.*, 1982). Spradlin and Siegel (1982) suggest that increasing children's motivation and their opportunities to use language may be the crucial elements in home-based training programmes, whilst Cheseldine and McConkey (1979) show that, at least for some parents, simply setting language goals may be sufficient to lead to considerable progress. For other families this is not enough and must be combined with specific training procedures. Again, the linguistic and social competence of the child is likely to be important and different types of strategy may well be required according to the child's level of development. For more responsive children who are already beginning to develop simple communicative skills, advice which helps parents to focus on the general development of language may be all that is required. The child's innate language competence will then be sufficient to guarantee progress. On the other hand, for children with very limited language ability, more highly structured programmes requiring a high degree of consistency in the use of prompting, modelling and reinforcement may be required to establish very simple linguistic rules.

Parental Competence

The importance of parental levels of competence for successful outcome has received little investigation. Clarke, Baker and Heifitz (1981) found that, in contrast with other studies of home intervention (Rinn, Vernon and Wise, 1975; Sandler, Seydon, Howe and Kaminsky, 1976), educational levels and socioeconomic skills were closely related to short-term progress. However, these factors did not predict longer-term results. The degree of parent co-operation during training was far more likely to predict their eventual competence in using behavioural techniques. The authors were not able to predict which parents would prove most co-operative but with additional training it was possible to increase proficiency, even amongst less involved parents. Unfortunately, children's performances were not necessarily found to be related to parental skills!

Sajwaj (1973) found that high levels of co-operation are not enough to predict outcome and, even with the most co-operative of families, programmes may fail unless they are tailored to existing domestic circumstances (which may well change with time) and to the needs of the particular child. Gray and Wandersman (1980) also suggest that there are many other variables relating to family life which may affect outcome, such as levels of father participation, mother's health, numbers of siblings, and the relationship between therapist and family, and Kessen and Fein (1975) found that mothers with large supportive networks were more receptive to home-based intervention. None of these studies examine outcome in terms of linguistic development and on the whole their findings are only suggestive of factors which *might* relate to children's progress.

The association between children's language ability and the verbal stimulation they receive from parents is also in need of further investigation. Howlin (1979) examined the relationshp between changes in the speech of autistic children and parents' use of language-directed utterances (viz., prompts, reinforcements, corrections, imitations and expansions). Increases in the general *frequency* of parents' utterances to their chilren were not related to improvements in children's speech, but alterations in parents' *style* of communication were associated with increases in children's speech. Unfortunately, although it is tempting to speculate that changes in parents' speech (following home intervention) were responsible for improvements in their children's language, this relationship was not experimentally investigated, and judgements about causality, based on correlational studies, must obviously remain highly tentative. In fact, in most cases the relationship is probably a highly complex one, with, perhaps, linguistic training by parents being responsible for some initial increases in children's use of speech. As the child's communication grows, however, this may then influence parents' responsiveness — leading then to greater communication by their children.

Summary

Unhappily, it seems that this review of language intervention leaves more questions unanswered than answered. In general, it appears that parents can be trained as language therapists. It is also apparent that intervention based at home rather than in the laboratory does not preclude the use of relatively sophisticated experimental manipulations nor or reliable assessment measures. Evidence from individual case studies suggests that home-based language training is effective with some children, and there is some information available regarding the types of chidren who are most likely to respond to treatment. However, we still know relatively little about which aspects of training are most important for outcome. Neither do we know how the child's developmental level may be related to these various training procedures. Individual differences in parents' competence and the relationships between children's ability levels and the teaching skills of their families have also to be explored. Assessment measures, too, need to be modified in order to ensure that they are more sensitive to changes in language development.

Home-based intervention is not an easy mode of research. As Gray and Wandersman (1980) point out, it is neither possible, nor desirable, to design a perfectly controlled experiment in which real people are assigned to treatment 'cells' and tested for 'effect'. Home-based programmes need to come to terms with the inevitable variations among children and their interactions with the environment, and we need to go beyond looking for significant differences between groups on narrowly defined outcomes. Instead, the effects of treatment for different subgroups of children need to be further explored, not only in terms of their language development but in terms of social and behavioural outcomes, too. No one study is likely to achieve all this, and it is unrealistic to expect any single investigation to answer all the remaining questions. Instead, several separate, but co-ordinated, studies, looking systematically into the effects of different aspects of treatment with children at differing levels of IQ and language, are needed. Such a consortium of studies would, hopefully, answer far more questions about the effects of language therapy than the large numbers of unconnected and frequently poorly controlled single case or small group studies currently in existence can ever do. However, even if the time or funds are not available to carry out more complex research, individual case or small group studies could still do far more to answer the questions posed by this review if they were to follow, more closely, the basic requirements of experimental research.

References

Attwood, T. (1977a) The Priory Parents Workshop, *Child: Care Health and Development, 3*, 81-91
——-(1977b) The Croydon Workshop for Pre-school Children, unpublished report, Croydon Social Services Dept.
Barnes, S., Gutfreund, M., Sattersly, D. and Wells, G. (1983) Characteristics of adult speech which predict children's language development, *Journal of Child Language, 10*, 65-84
Bennett, C.W. (1973) A four and a half year old as a teacher of her hearing impaired sister: A case study, *Journal of Communication Disorders, 6*, 67-75
Berkowitz, B.P. and Graziano, A.M. (1972) Training parents as behaviour therapists: a review, *Behaviour Research and Therapy, 10*, 197-317
Bloch, J., Gersten, E. and Kornblum, J. (1980) Evaluation of a language program for young autistic children, *Journal of Speech and Hearing Disorders, 45*, 76-89
Bidder, R., Bryant, G. and Gray, O. (1975) Benefits to Down's Syndrome children through training their mothers, *Archives of Disorders of Childhood, 50*, 383-6
Brasel, K. and Quigley, S. (1977) Influences of certain language and communication environments in early childhood on the development of language in deaf individuals, *Journal of Speech and Hearing Research, 20*, 93-107
Brown, R. (1973) *A First Language: The Early Stages*, George Allen and Unwin, London
——and Hanlon, C. (1970) Derivational complexity and order of acquisition in child speech, in J.R. Hayes (ed.), *Cognition and the Development of Language*, Wiley, New York
Buium, N., Rynders, J. and Turnure, J. (1974) Early maternal linguistic environment of normal and Down's Syndrome language learning children, *American Journal of Mental Deficiency, 79*, 52-8
Callias, M. (1980) Teaching parents, teachers and nurses, in W. Yule and J. Carr (eds.), *Behaviour Modification for the Mentally Handicapped*, Croom Helm, London

Cambell, D.T. and Stanley, J.C. (1966) *Experimental and Quasi Experimental Designs for Research*, Rand McNally, Chicago

Cantwell, D., Howlin, P. and Rutter, M. (1977) The analysis of language level and language function, *British Journal of Disorders of Communication, 12*, 119-35

Carpenter, R.L. and Augustine, L.E. (1973) A pilot training programme for parent clinicians, *Journal of Speech and Hearing Disorders, 38*, 48-58

Carrier, J. (1970) A program of articulation therapy administered by mothers, *Journal of Speech and Hearing Disorders, 35*, 344-8

Casey, L.O. (1978) Development of communicative behavior in autistic children: A parent program using manual signs, *Journal of Autism and Childhood Schizophrenia, 8*, 45-59

Cazden, C. (1965) Envionmental Assistance to the Child's Acquisition of Grammar, unpublished doctoral dissertation, University of Harvard

Cheseldine, S. and McConkey, R. (1979) Parental speech to young Down's Syndrome children: An intervention study, *American Journal of Mental Deficiency, 83*, 612-20

Clarke, D., Baker, B. and Heifitz, L. (1981) Behavioral training for parents of mentally retarded children: Prediction and Outcome, *American Journal of Mental Deficiency, 86*, 14-19

Clarke-Stewart, K.A. (1973) Interactions between mothers and their young children: Characteristics and Consequences, *Monographs of the Society for Research in Child Development, 38*, Nos. 6-7, Serial No. 153

Clements, J., Bidder, R., Gardner, S., Bryant, G. and Gray, O. (1980) A home advisory service for pre-school children with developmental delays, *Child: Care Health and Development, 6*, 25-33

——Evans, C., Jones, C., Osborne, K. and Upton, G. (1982) Evaluation of a home based language training programme with severely mentally handicapped children, *Behaviour Research and Therapy, 20*, 243-9

Cooper, J., Moodley, M. and Reynell, J. (1979) The developmental language programme. Results from a five year study, *British Journal of Disorders of Communication, 14*, 57-69

Cross, T.G. (1977) Mothers' speech adjustments: the contribution of selected child listener variables, in C. Snow and C. Ferguson (eds.), *Talking to Children: Language Input and Acquisition*, University of Cambridge Press, Cambridge

Cunningham, C., Reuler, E., Blackwell, J. and Deck, J. (1981) Behavioral and linguistic developments in the interactions of normal and retarded children with their mothers, *Child Development, 52*, 62-70

Davis, A. (1947) Some experiences with two small groups of mothers in a child guidance clinic, *British Journal of Psychiatric Social Work, 1*, 16-22

Eysenck, H.J. (1961) The Effects of Psychotherapy, in H.J. Eysenck (ed.), *Handbook of Abnormal Psychology*, Basic Books, New York

Farwell, C. (1973) The language spoken to children, *Papers and Reports on Child Language Development No. 5*, 31-62, Stanford University, Stanford

Feldman, C. (1970) The Effects of Various Types of Adult Responses in the Syntactic Acquisition of Two to Three Year-olds, unpublished report, University of Chicago

Forehand, R., Guest, D. and Weil, K. (1979) Parent behavioral training: An analysis of the relationship among multiple outcome measures, *Journal of Abnormal Child Psychology, 4*, 229-42

Frank, S., Allen, D., Stein, L. and Meyrs, B. (1976) Linguistic performance in vulnerable and autistic children and their mothers, *American Journal of Psychiatry, 133*, 909-15

Furrow, D., Nelson, K. and Benedict, H. (1979) Mothers' speech to children and syntactic development: Some simple relationships, *Journal of Child Language, 6*, 423-42

Garcia, E. and De Haven, E.D. (1974) Use of operant techniques in the establishment and generalisation of language: A review and analysis, *American Journal of Mental Deficiency, 79*, 169-78

———and Wallace, M.B. (1977) Parental training of the plural morpheme in normal toddlers, *Journal of Behavior Analysis, 10*, 505

Gardner, J. (1969) Behavior modification research in mental retardation: Search for an adequate paradigm, *American Journal of Mental Deficiency, 73*, 844-51

———Pearson, D.T., Bercovici, N. and Bricker, D.D. (1968) Measurement, evaluation, and modification of selected social interactions between a schizophrenic child, his parents and his therapist, *Journal of Consulting and Clinical Psychology, 32*, 537-42

Gath, A. (1979) Parents as therapists of mentally handicapped children, *Journal of Child Psychology and Psychiatry, 20*, 161-6

Gerber, A. and Goehl, H. (1980) The Temple University Short Syntax Test, unpublished manuscript, Phildadelphia, Temple University. Cited in A. Gerber and D.N. Bryen (eds.), *Language and Learning Disabilities*, University Park Press, Baltimore

Goldstein, S.B. and Lanyon, R.I. (1971) Parent clinicians in the language training of an autistic child, *Journal of Speech and Hearing Disorders, 36*, 552-60

Gray, S. and Wandersman, L. (1980) The methodology of home based intervention studies: Problems and promising strategies, *Child Development, 31*, 993-1009

Hamblin, R.L., Buckholdt, D., Ferritor, D., Kozloff, M. and Blackwell, L. (1971) *The Humanization Processes: A Social, Behavioral Analysis of Children's Problems*, John Wiley, New York

Harris, S.L. (1975) Language to non-verbal children with emphasis on problems of generalisation, *Psychological Bulletin, 82*, 565-80

———and Wolchick, S. (1982) Speech skills to non-verbal children and their parents, in J. Steffen and P. Karoly (eds.), *Autism and Severe Psychopathology: Advances in Child Behavioral Analysis and Therapy*, Vol. 2, D.C. Heaton, Lexington

———Wolchik, S. and Weiss, S. (1981) The acquisition of language skills by autistic children: Can parents do the job? *Journal of Autism and Developmental Disorders, 11*, 373-84

Hawkins, R.P., Peterson, R.C., Schweid, E. and Bijou, S.W. (1966) Behavior therapy in the home: Amelioration of problem parent-child relations with the parent in a therapeutic role, *Journal of Experimental Child Psychology, 4*, 99-107

Hemsley, R., Howlin, P., Berger, M., Hersov, L., Holbrook, D., Rutter, M. and Yule, W. (1978) Treating autistic children in a family context, in M. Rutter and E. Schopler (eds.), *Autism: Reappraisal of Concepts and Treatment*, Plenum , New York

Hislop, M.W. (1971) Behavioral management services for the retarded: Application of operant training procedures in the home, *Ontario Psychologist, 3*, 1-12

Holmes, N., Hemsley, R., Rickett, J. and Likierman, H. (1982) Parents as co-therapists: Their perceptions of a home based behavioural treatment for autistic children, *Journal of Autism and Developmental Disorders, 12*, 331-42

Horner, R. and Baer, D. (1978) Multiple-probe techniques: A variation of the multiple baseline, *Journal of Applied Behavior Analysis, 11*, 189-96

Howe, C. (1981) *Acquiring Language in a Conversational Context*, Academic Press, London

Howlin, P. (1979) Training Parents to Modify the Language of their Autistic

Children: A Home Based Approach, unpublished Ph.D. thesis, University of London

—— (1980a) The home treatment of autistic children, in L.A. Hersov, M. Berger and R. Nichol (eds.), *Language and Language Disorders in Children*, Pergamon, Oxford

—— (1980b) Language training with the severely retarded, in W. Yule and J. Carr (eds.), *Behaviour Modification with the Severely Retarded*, Croom Helm, London

—— (1981a) The effectiveness of operant language training with autistic children, *Journal of Autism and Developmental Disorders, 11*, 89-105

—— (1981b) The results of a home-based language training programme with autistic children, *British Journal of Disorders of Communication, 16*, 21-9

Hursh, D.E. and Sherman, J.A. (1973) The effects of parent presented models and praise on the behavior of their children, *Journal of Experimental Child Psychology, 7*, 328-39

Jeffree, D.M. and Cashdan, A. (1971) Severely subnormal children and their parents: an experiment in language improvement, *British Journal of Educational Psychology, 41*, 184-94

—— Wheldall, K. and Mittler, D. (1973) Facilitating two-word utterances in two Down's Syndrome boys, *American Journal of Mental Deficiency, 78*, 117-22

Johnson, C.A. and Katz, R.C. (1973) Using parents as change agents for their children: A review, *Journal of Child Psychology and Psychiatry, 14*, 181-200

Johnson, S. and Brown, R. (1969) Producing behavior change in parents of disturbed children, *Journal of Child Psychology and Psychiatry, 10*, 107-21

Jones, C., Clements, J., Evans, C., Osborne, K. and Upton, G. (1983) South Wales Early Language Research project, *Mental Handicap, 11*, 30-32

Kaufman, K. and Kozloff, M. (1977) New Directions in Comprehensive Programming for Parents of Autistic Children, Application and Evaluation of 'Kozloff-Type' Parent Training Program, Sagmore Children's Centre

Kaye, K. and Charney, R. (1981) Conversational asymmetry between mothers and children, *Journal of Child Language, 8*, 35-50

Kazdin, A.E. (1973a) Methodological and assessment considerations in evaluating reinforcement programs in applied settings, *Journal of Applied Behavior Analysis, 6*, 517-31

—— (1973b) Issues in behavior modification with mentally retarded persons, *American Journal of Mental Deficiency, 78*, 134-40

Kessen, W. and Fein, G. (1975) *Variations in Home-Based Infant Education: Language Play and Social Development*, Yale University Press, New Haven

Koegel, R., Glahn, T. and Nieminen, G. (1978) Generalisation of parent training results, *Journal of Applied Behavior Analysis, 11*, 95-109

—— Rincover, A. and Egel, A. (eds.) (1982) *Educating and Understanding Autistic Children*, College Press, Houston

Kogan, K.L. and Tyler, N. (1973) Mother-child interaction in young, physically handicapped children, *American Journal of Mental Deficiency, 77*, 492-7

Kozloff, M.A. (1973) *Reaching the Autistic Child: A Parent Training Program*, Research Press, Champaign, Illinois

Lazky, E. and Klopp, K. (1982) Parent child interactions in normal and language disordered children, *Journal of Speech and Hearing Disorders, 47*, 7-18

Levenstein, P. (1971) Mother-child home program, *Childhood Education, 43*, 130-4

Lieven, E. (1978) Conversation between mothers and young children: Individual differences and their possible implications for the study of language learning, in N. Waterson and C. Snow (eds.), *The Development of Communication: Social, and Pragmatic Factors in Language Acquisition*, Wiley, London

Lombardino, L. and Magnan N. (1983) Parents as language trainers: language programming with developmentally delayed children, *Exceptional Children, 49*, 358-61

Lovaas, O.I. (1966) A program for the establishment of speech in psychotic children, in J.K. Wing (ed.), *Early Childhood Autism: Clinical, Educational and Social Aspects*, Pergamon, Oxford

——(1977a) Parents as therapists for autistic children, in M. Rutter and E. Schopler (eds.), *Autism: Reappraisal of Concepts and Treatment*, Plenum, New York

——(1977b) *The Autistic Child: Language Development Through Behavior Modification*, Wiley, New York

——Koegel, R., Simmons, J. and Stevens, J. (1973) Some generalisation and follow-up measures on autistic children in behaviour therapy, *Journal of Applied Behavior Analysis, 6*, 131-66

McConkey, R., Jeffree, D. and Hewson, S. (1979) Involving parents in extending the language development of their young mentally handicapped children, *British Journal of Disorders of Communication, 14*, 203-19

McDonagh, T.S. and McNamara, J.R. (1973) Design-criteria relationships in behavior therapy with children, *Journal of Child Psychology and Psychiatry, 14*, 271-82

MacDonald, J.D., Blott, J.P., Gordon, K., Spiegel, B. and Hartmann, M. (1974) An experimental parent assisted treatment program for preschool language delayed children, *Journal of Speech and Hearing Disorders, 39*, 395-415

Marshall, N.R., Hegrenes, J.R. and Goldstein, S. (1973) Verbal interactions: Mothers and their retarded children vs. mothers and their non-retarded chidren, *American Journal of Mental Deficiency, 77*, 415-9

Mash, E. and Terdal, L. (1973) Modification of mother-child interaction playing with children, *Mental Retardation, 10*, 44-9

Mathis, M.I. (1971) Training of a 'disturbed' boy using the mother as therapist: A case study, *Behavior Therapy, 2*, 233-9

Miller, S. and Sloane, M. (1976) The generalization effects of parent training across stimulus settings, *Journal of Applied Behavior Analysis, 9*, 355-70

Moerk, E.L. (1972) Principles of interaction in language training, *Merrill Palmer Quarterly, 19*, 229-57

Munro, D. (1952) An experiment in the use of group methods with parents in a child guidance clinic, *British Journal of Psychiatric Social Work, 6*, 16-20

Nelson, K. (1973) Structure and strategy in learning to talk, *Monographs of the Society for Research in Child Development, 38*, 1-2, Serial No. 149

——(1977) Facilitating children's syntax acquisition, *Developmental Psychology, 13*, 101-7

——(1981) Individual differences in language development: Implications for development and language, *Developmental Psychology, 17*, 170-87

Newport, E. Gleitman, H. and Gleitman, L. (1977) Mother, I'd rather do it myself: Some effects and non effects of maternal speech style, in C. Snow and C. Feignan (eds.), *Talking to Children*, Cambridge University Press, Cambridge

Nolan, J.D. and Pence, C. (1970) Operant conditioning principles in the treatment of a selectively mute child, *Journal of Consulting and Clinical Psychology, 35*, 265-8

Nordquist, V.M. and Wahler, R.G. (1973) Naturalistic treatment of an autistic child, *Journal of Applied Behavior Analysis, 6*, 79-87

O'Dell, S. (1974) Training parents in behavior modification: A review, *Psychological Bulletin, 81*, 418-33

Olsen-Fulero, L. (1982) Style and stability of mother conversational behaviour: a study of individual differences, *Journal of Child Language, 9*, 563-6

Palmer, H. and Anderson, L. (1980) Long term gains from early intervention: Findings from longitudinal studies, in E. Zigler and J. Valentine (eds.), *Project Headstart: A Legacy of the War on Poverty*, The Free Press, New York

Park, D. (1974) Operant conditioning of a speaking autistic child, *Journal of Autism and Childhood Schizophrenia, 4*, 189-90

Pawlicki, R. (1970) Behavior-therapy research with children: a critical review, *Canadian Journal of Behavioral Sciences, 2*, 163-75

Peterson, G. and Sherrod, K. (1982) Relationships of maternal language to language development and language delay in children, *American Journal of Mental Deficiency, 4*, 391-8

Prutting, C.A., Gallagher, T. and Mulac, A. (1975) The expressive portion of the N.S.S.T. compared to a spontaneous language sample, *Journal of Speech and Hearing Disorders, 40*, 40-8

Raver, S., Cooke, T. and Apolloni, T. (1978) Generalization effects from intra therapy articulation training: A case study, *Journal of Applied Behavior Analysis, 11*, 436

Revill, S. and Blunden, R. (1979) A home-training service for pre-school developmentally handicapped children, *Behaviour Research and Therapy, 17*, 207-14

Rhine, W. (ed.) (1981) *Making Schools More Effective: New Directions from Follow Through*, Academic Press, New York

Rinn, R., Vernon, J. and Wise, M. (1975) Training parents of behaviorally disordered children in groups: A 3 years' program evaluation, *Behavior Therapy, 6*, 378-87

Risley, T.R. and Baer, D.M. (1973) Operant behavior modification: The deliberate development of behavior, in B.C. Caldwell and H.N. Ricciuti (eds.), *Review of Child Development Research: 3. Child Development and Social Policy*, University of Chicago Press, Chicago

Rondal, J. (1978) Maternal speech to normal and Down's Syndrome children matched for mean length of utterance, in C.E. Meyers (ed.), *Quality of Life in Severly and Profoundly Mentally Retarded People*, Research Foundations for Improvement, American Association on Mental Deficiencies Monograph 3, Washington DC

Rose, S. (1976) Group training of parents as behavior modifiers, *Social Work, 19*, 156-62

Routh, D. (1969) Conditioning vocal response differentiation in infants, *Developmental Psychology, 1*, 219-26

Russo, S. (1964) Adaptations in behaviour therapy with children, *Behaviour Research and Therapy, 2*, 43-7

Rutter, M. (1980) Language training with autistic children: How does it work and What does it achieve?, in L.A. Hersov, M. Berger and R. Nichol (eds.), *Language and Language Disorders in Children*, Pergamon, Oxford

Sajwaj, T. (1973) Difficulties in the use of behavioral techniques by parents in changing child behavior: Guides to success, *Journal of Nervous and Mental Disorders, 156*, 395-403

Salvin, A., Routh, D., Foster, R.E. and Lovejoy, K. (1977) Acquisition of modified American sign language by a mute autistic child, *Journal of Autism and Childhood Schizophrenia, 7*, 359-71

Salzburg, C. and Villani, T. (1983) Speech training by parents of Down's Syndrome toddlers: Generalisation across settings and instructional contexts, *American Journal of Mental Deficiency, 4*, 403-13

Sandler, A., Coren, A. and Thurman, S. (1983) A training program for parents of handicapped children: Effects upon mother, father and child, *Exceptional Children, 49*, 355-7

Sandler, O., Seydon, T., Howe, B. and Kaminsky, T. (1976) An evaluation of

'Groups for Parents': A standardized format encompassing both behavior modification and humanistic methods, *Journal of Community Psychology, 4*, 157-63

Sandow, S., Clarke, A., Cox, M. and Stewart, F. (1981) Home intervention with parents of severely subnormal pre-school children: A final report, *Child: Care Health and Development, 7*, 135-55

Schiff, N. (1979) The influence of deviant maternal speech on the development of language during the pre-school years, *Journal of Speech and Hearing Research, 22*, 581-601

Schopler, E. and Reichler, R.J. (1971) Developmental therapy by parents with their own autistic child, in M.L. Rutter (ed.), *Infantile Autism: Concepts, Characteristics and Treatment*, Churchill Livingstone, Edinburgh

Seitz, S. and Hoekenger, R. (1974) Modeling as a training tool for retarded children and their parents, *Mental Retardation, 12*, No. 2, 28-9

——and Marcus, S. (1976) Mother-child interactions: A formulation for language development, *Exceptional Children, 43*, 23-6

Shatz, M. (1982) On mechanisms of language acquisition: Can features of the communication environment account for development?, in E. Warner and L. Gleitman (eds.), *Language Acquisition: The State of the Art*, Cambridge University Press, Cambridge

Shelton, R., Johnson, A., Ruscello, D. and Arndt, W. (1978) Assessment of parent administered listening training for pre-school children with articulation deficits, *Journal of Speech and Hearing Disorders, 43*, 242-53

Sherman, J.A. and Baer, D.M. (1968) Appraisal of operant techniques with children and adults, in C.M. Franks (ed.), *Behavior Therapy: Appraisal and Status*, McGraw Hill, New York

Sloane, H.N. and MacAulay, B.D. (1968) *Operant Procedures in Remedial Speech and Language Training*, Houghton Mifflin, Boston

Snow, C.E. (1977) The Development of Conversation between mothers and babies, *Journal of Child Language, 4*, 1-22

——and Ferguson, C. (1977) *Talking to Children: Language Input and Acquisition*, Cambridge University Press, Cambridge

Spradlin, J. and Siegel, G. (1982) Language training in natural and clinical environments, *Journal of Speech and Hearing Disorders, 47*, 2-6

Stevenson, P., Bax, M. and Stevenson, J. (1982) The evaluation of home based speech therapy for language delayed pre-school children in an inner city area, *British Journal of Disorders of Communication, 17*, 141-8

Terdal, L., Brose, D., Buell, J., Busch, S. and Cheledin, L. (1969a), unpublished laboratory manual, University of Oregon Medical School

——and Buell, J. (1969b) Parent education in managing retarded children with behavior deficits and inappropriate behaviors, *Mental Retardation, 7*, 10-13

Tharp, R. and Wetzel, R. (1969) *Behavior Modification in the Natural Environment*, Academic Press, New York

Van Kleek, A. and Carpenter, R. (1980) The effects of children's language comprehension level on adults' child-directed talk, *Journal of Speech and Hearing Research, 23*, 546-70

Vorster, J. (1975) Mommy linguist: The case for motherese, *Lingua, 37*, 281-312

Welsh, R.S. (1966) A Highly Efficient Method of Parental Counselling, Paper presented at the Rocky Mountain Psychological Association, cited in B. Berkowitz and A. Graziano (1972), Training parents as behavior therapists: A review, *Behaviour Research and Therapy, 10*, 297-317

Whitehurst, G.J., Novak, G. and Zorn, G.A. (1972) Delayed speech studied in the home, *Developmental Psychology, 7*, 169-77

Williams, C. (1959) The elimination of tantrum behavior by extinction procedures, *Journal of Abnormal and Social Psychology, 59*, 269-71

Wolchick, S. and Harris, S. (1982) Language environments of autistic and normal children matched for language age: A preliminary investigation, *Journal of Autism and Developmental Disorders, 12*, 43-55

Wolf, M., Risley, T., Johnston, M., Harris, F. and Allen, E. (1967) Application of operant conditioning procedures to the behaviour problems of an autistic child: A follow-up and extension, *Behaviour Research and Therapy, 5*, 103-11

—— Risley, T.R. and Mees, H.I. (1964) Applications of operant conditioning procedures to the behaviour problems of an autistic child, *Behaviour Research and Therapy, 2*, 305-12

Yule, W. (1974) Single case studies methodology in the evaluation of therapeutic intervention, Paper read to the 9th International Study Group on Child Neurology and Cerebral Palsy, Oxford, September

—— (1975) Teaching psychological principles to non psychologists: Training parents in child management, *Journal of the Association of Educational Psychologists, 10*, 5-16

—— and Berger, M. (1975) Communication, language, and behaviour modification, in C. Kiernan and F. Woodward (eds.), *Behaviour Modification with the Severely Retarded*, Associated Scientific Publications, Amsterdam

Zigler, E. and Valentine, J. (1980) *Project Head Start: A Legacy of the War on Poverty*, The Free Press, New York

10 TEACHING CHILDREN TO DEVELOP LANGUAGE: THE IMPOSSIBLE DREAM?

John Harris

In spite of the recent concern for translating developments in linguistic theory into practical recommendations for language training, and the proliferation of language teaching schemes designed to improve the linguistic abilities of language-disordered children, professionals involved in language therapy have met with little success in their efforts to provide clear guidelines for language instruction. An examination of the recent work in the field of language intervention indicates two types of response to this unfortunate state of affairs. Firstly, there are those who look toward the linguistic theories which have served as the bases for the derivation of a developmental sequence of learning objectives within different teaching schemes; as linguistic descriptions have become more elaborate and extensive, so there have been systematic attempts to broaden the language teaching curriculum. For example, whereas 20 years ago under the influence of Chomskian grammatical descriptions of adult language, the majority of language schemes sought to teach linguistic structures, more recent schemes have sought to include specification of desirable semantic features and pragmatic/functional characteristics. (For a useful review of this approach see McLean and Snyder-McLean, Chapter 3).

The second type of reaction to the failure of language instruction programmes arises from the fact that many intervention studies have reported considerable difficulty in achieving generalisation of skills, attained during the training sessions, to other more natural contexts. This has prompted some psychologists to question the clinical model of intervention whereby individual children are seen by a specially trained therapist in a clinical setting. It has been suggested that the child's difficulty lies in transferring a skill acquired in one setting with one individual, to other individuals in other contexts. In order to overcome this problem teachers and parents have been encouraged to teach language to children within familiar everyday settings in the expectation that the difference between the training context and naturally occurring situations for language use will be reduced and hence more easily bridged by the child (MacDonald, Blott, Gordon, Spiegel and

Hartmann, 1974; Mahoney, 1975; Seitz, 1975; Mahoney, Crawley and Pullis, 1980).

One assumption which is characteristic of all language teaching schemes is that the sequence of abilities which spontaneously *develop* in normal children, can be established in language disordered children by direct instruction, and it is suggested that the absence of a clear conceptual distinction between the two processes lies at the heart of the failure of language intervention schemes. It is not simply that those concerned with the design of intervention schemes have lacked an adequate description of what language is, nor that psychologists have adopted inappropriate teaching strategies; the problem lies in the mistaken belief that it is somehow possible to bypass development and yet achieve attainments which are indistinguishable from natural developmental products.

What is Meant by Development?

Shotter (1982) has recently pointed out the significance of the scientist's 'background talk' if one wishes to arrive at an understanding of the implicit model which gives rise to specific research questions and constitutes the basis for interpretation of results. In order to understand properly the inherent contradictions of attempts to teach language development, it is necessary to consider the different ways in which psychologists talk about and understand the term 'development', and assumptions which lie behind the use of the word 'teaching', in the context of intervention strategies. Francis (1980) has suggested three popular interpretations of the term development.

(i) Development may be accorded an intransitive meaning, incorporating ideas of growth, evolution and maturation. For example, 'that little boy is developing very rapidly'. Such an interpretation is consistent with Chomsky's view of the emergence of language (Chomsky, 1965) but it provides very little guidance in relation to possible language intervention strategies; there is no way of rewiring a damaged language acquisition device.

(ii) Development may receive a transitive interpretation which implies building or elaborating some *thing* (e.g. the child is slow/ needs help in developing language). This is congruent with the notion of language being an acquired skill and the Skinnerian view that language should be subject to direct modification by the manipulation of environmental contingencies (Skinner, 1957).

(iii) Development is seen as characterising the emergence of new and unpredictable outcomes and is consistent with the notion of human development as a complex series of dialectical exchanges or transactions between the organism and the environment (Sameroff, 1975).

The vast amount of research which is currently being directed at language learning among normal children bears witness to how little is understood of this aspect of development and how limited is the psychologist's ability to predict outcomes, whether in respect of the sequence of words and sentences which constitutes a conversation or with regard to the precise course of language development in any individual child. In the case of language development, ignorance forces us to recognise the validity of Francis' third interpretation. However, development generally evokes an entirely different interpretation when applied to language-disordered children; either the first interpretation is apparent, in which case successful intervention is regarded as impossible, or the second meaning provides a conceptual base for language instruction.

The different meanings which are attributed to the term development in these two contexts are thrown into sharp relief when one considers that the role of normal children in language research is to be observed in order that psychologists might be informed about the nature of development. In contrast, children with language disorders are frequently exposed to procedures designed to influence what develops. The question of whether normal children might be subjected to systematic intervention procedures in order to influence the course of development never arises, because such a course of action is incompatible with a view of development as an unpredictable and inevitable unfolding of novel outcomes.

Furthermore, language teaching for language-disordered children only makes sense so long as the interpretation of the word 'development' which is applied to this group differs from the meaning usually ascribed to 'development' among normal children. It is argued below that teaching can make a contribution to the development of skills and abilities which *can* be clearly specified in advance of intervention (Francis' second meaning of the term 'development') but that teaching is incompatible with the notion of development as the emergence of new and unpredictable outcomes.

What is Involved in Teaching?

A second problem with regard to nomenclature concerns what is meant by the term 'teaching'. In attempting to clarify this concept Hirst (1973) emphasises the intentions of both the teacher and the pupil; the teacher must intend to teach something and must achieve this by establishing in the pupil the intention to learn. Teaching may be said to have occurred when the teacher is successful in bringing about in the pupil the desire to know, understand or master that which the teacher has deemed to be the content of the lesson.

Hirst's view, that teaching must begin with an analysis of the desired outcomes or changes in the pupils, is reflected in the status accorded to the curriculum in ordinary schools and also in the structure of the majority of language teaching programmes which psychologists and others have designed to promote the language of handicapped or developmentally delayed children. An increased concern among educators for accountability in education and among psychologists for direct measures of association between what is taught and what is learned, has resulted in widespread acceptance of the doctrine that intended outcomes ought to be specified in terms of behavioural objectives.

Within this framework, teaching can be described in terms of the specification of a curriculum which includes (or can be translated into) descriptions of target behaviour and the sequence in which elements within the curriculum should be presented, and secondly a delivery system or training technology which consists of the procedures for establishing the behaviours defined by the curriculum (Ruder, 1978; Mahoney, Crawley and Pullis, 1980). It is this model of teaching which has been most frequently embraced, either implicitly or explicitly, by the designers of language development teaching programmes and it is this model which I propose to criticise as being inconsistent with contemporary knowledge of language devloment (Miller and Yoder, 1972, 1974; Muma, 1977; Leeming, Swann, Coupe and Mittler, 1979; Gillham, 1979, 1982).

Problems of Trying to Teach Children to Develop Language

To the extent that the goal of language intervention is to assist the language-disordered child to achieve, as far as is possible, the same abilities as normal children, that is control of a natural language and not an artificial and strictly circumscribed set of language-like responses, then it is possible to criticise teaching approaches on two counts; the first is concerned with the limitations of the curriculum and the second is concerned with the processes which characterise formal instruction.

Any attempt to devise a language curriculum as a basis for the setting up of teaching objectives and evaluating the effectiveness of intervention will have the following limitations.

(i) Language curricula are based on descriptions which have emerged from observation and experimental work with one population (i.e. normal children). They are then applied to a totally different population, although there is little empirical evidence to indicate that the dictum of 'slow but normal language development' among language disordered groups is valid.

(ii) Curricula are based on summary language data from a large number of children from different cultures and, to the extent that research in the last two decades has concentrated upon a search for inter-individual regularities during development, it has underrated the range of individual differences (Nelson, 1973, 1980). For this reason group data cannot provide an appropriate source of information for individual intervention.

(iii) The extent of the inter-individual variation among language-disordered children makes it extremely unlikely that the sequence of learning steps will be identical for different individuals. On the other hand there are simply no empirical and theoretical guidelines available to suggest how a general curriculum might be modified to suit individuals.

(iv) Recent history indicates that descriptions of human language have been subjected to continuous elaborations and modifications (e.g. Lock, 1980) and there is no reason to believe that this process is likely to come to an end. Such descriptions are therefore bound to provide incomplete and distorted characterisations of normal language development.

(v) Children do not, and probably cannot, learn a first language as an object in itself, since it is only by participating in language games with others that they can come to understand what language is. If language is in a sense a by-product of the child's striving for functional control of the social world, it is illogical to expect the recipient of early language intervention to participate in the exercise in the same way that a child who is being taught to read or to play the piano participates by sharing with the teacher an understanding of what it is that is trying to be achieved. To the extent that language development occurs accidentally, or at least without any intention on the part of the child to learn language, it will not be amenable to replication in language-disordered children by teaching.

A teaching strategy is inappropriate to language development since teaching and development presuppose an entirely different relationship between the individual and the environment. Whereas teaching suggests that the environment may have a simple and direct effect on the learning products which may be established, development is considered to be the result of a complex set of transactions between the organism and the environment such that each influences and is influenced by the other. Any attempt to apply direct instruction to developmental processes gives rise to the following contradictions.

(i) In teaching there is no necessary connection between *what* is taught and *how* this might be achieved. Once objectives have been defined it is assumed that they can provide a clear guide to the selection and planning of learning experiences. Principles of human learning may be given prominence in such planning, but it is assumed that such principles are sufficiently general to be applied to any set of objectives. Thus, in teaching, the desired products of an interaction between the child and the environment are used to determine the processes which might be employed; in the case of human development the converse occurs — the processes are seen as determining the outcomes.

(ii) Since developmental outcomes do not bear any simple relationship to environmental inputs, attainments will be largely unpredictable; where intervention is successful in maintaining control of outcomes these will not be developmentally progressive but lower order associations between specific stimuli and responses. Such responses bear little relationship to natural language abilities (Rees, 1978). On the other hand, to the extent that natural language develops in spite of formal instruction, the child's emerging abilities will *not* be easily related to the teaching input.

(iii) Since teaching assumes external control over the products of instruction, such an approach is antagonistic to one of the main characteristics of natural language — spontaneity. Just as formal instruction cannot cope with development as the manifestation of unexpected outcomes, so it is incapable of specifying and teaching the flexibility and novelty which typifies everyday speech of children and adult alike.

(iv) If the basis of linguistic skill is seen as some form of knowledge or competence, then another problem for an instructional approach to first language learning becomes apparent. When teaching skills or behaviours, information regarding successful learning is provided by the subject's response – appropriate responses indicate successful learning while variations from the optimal goal behaviour may provide information relevant to subsequent training. Using this approach to teach cognitive representations – or the knowledge which underlies language performance – relies upon two untested assumptions: firstly, that it is possible to establish a direct link between a particular underlying cognitive representation and particular linguistic behaviours, and secondly, that the normal process by which competence and performance are related can be modified so that the exercise of skilled performance can become a basis for the generation of internal representations. But development involves a complex interplay of knowledge and the functional reinterpretation of that knowledge within a specific context, so that linguistic performance is influenced by an individual's knowledge as well as creating the possibility for further modifications and reorganisation of that knowledge (Ryan, 1973; Newson, 1979). Language teaching strategies are employed in the mistaken belief that the exercise of skilled performance, under the control of artificially manipulated environmental contingencies (and thus severed from the functional implications of natural language use), can itself become the sole basis for the generation of linguistic knowledge. There is thus a confusion between the methods which are appropriate for teaching *skills*, and the methods which can be used to facilitate the development of linguistic competence.

An Alternative Strategy

The contradictions which arise from the attempts to teach language development mean that language instruction inevitably involves conflict and compromise. To a greater or lesser degree, current language programmes ignore developmental processes and concentrate on establishing curriculum goals; the effect of this is to provide the child with skills which bear only a passing resemblance to natural language by employing strategies which may be inimical to natural development. The alternative would be for those concerned with intervention to abrogate language instruction and elect instead to *facilitate developmental pro-*

cesses. Effective developmentally-oriented intervention would require a shift by language therapists away from predictive curriculum-dominated models of intervention and toward an ecologically based process model, which would be concerned with the identification of those conditions which are maximally facilitative of language development among children of different ages, abilities and aetiologies, and descriptions of the social and communicative interactions involved. Mahoney (1975) has argued for an ecological approach to language intervention which would be consistent with what is known of the kinds of social and communicative interactions which underlie both pre-verbal and verbal communication among normal children. He advocated training adult models 'to synchronise their communication strategies with those of the children so that there would be a relatively efficient pre-verbal or non-verbal communication system between them' (p. 145). However, Mahoney described both appropriate and inappropriate communicative exchanges between adults and children as arising from the characteristics of the participants, irrespective of any situational constraints. A number of recent studies have shown that the characteristics of any adult-child interaction to be heavily influenced by variables such as the location, activity, materials available, purpose of the interaction, and physical proximity of adult and child (Fraser and Roberts, 1975; Dunn, Wooding and Hermann, 1977; Wood, MacMahon and Cranstoun, 1980; Tizard, Hughes, Carmichael, Pinkerton, 1983). Any attempt to replicate the characteristics of 'normal' adult and child interactions without taking account of these and other situational variables, would be retrogressive since it would inevitably lead back toward teaching superficial skills and behaviours with all the pitfalls described above.

Before developmentally-orientated intervention strategies can be considered, applied psychologists need to answer the following questions

(i) What are the activities and social interactions to which language-disordered children are exposed?

(ii) What communicative and linguistic interactions occur during those activities?

(iii) To what extent are there variations in the communicative interactions between and within situations?

For example, in a recent study by Harris (1982) it was found that young mentally handicapped children in a Special School were regularly involved in one-to-one language teaching sessions and also in loosely structured group activities. Detailed analysis of the verbal and non-verbal interactions indicated considerable variation over the two situations. In particular, there was a higher frequency of spontaneous initiations by the children, and a much higher proportion of appropriate compared to inappropriate responses to adult questions, in the unstructured situation. If one accepts these two measures as providing an index of the quality of language learning opportunities occurring in the two settings, the informal unstructured activity was more conducive to language development than the structured one-to-one language teaching session. In another study of mentally handicapped children, Brinker (1982) has shown that two symbolic play contexts differed regarding the extent to which children were able to name objects involved in situationally appropriate actions. He suggests that whereas the materials for putting a doll to bed involve actions and objects which are integrated around the concept of *baby*, a tea party situation involved a set of divergent or non-integrated action-object relations. On the basis of this interpretation, the 'putting dolly to bed' context was more easily integrated into a co-ordinated representational substrate for the lexical items. Eventually studies such as these might reverse the current state of knowledge in relation to language-disordered children, whereby psychologists and teachers know a great deal about the kinds of *instructional* approaches which *do not* succeed but very little about the natural ecology of language development among language-disordered groups.

The question remains of whether within an ecologically based developmental model it is possible to move from observation and description to intervention and prescription. There are two related obstacles to this transition. Firstly, if development is conceived as the unique unfolding of unpredictable potentialities, then any form of prescriptive intervention must be restricted to statements regarding the *general* features of communicative exchanges which are *likely* to be advantageous (Seibert and Kimbrough Oller, 1981). This limits the language clinician to making statements about the quality of interactions, in the belief that those interactions which are identified as being of 'high quality' will be more beneficial to language learning children than interactions which are regarded as 'low quality'.

However, the attempt to clarify interactions in terms of quality highlights the second difficulty, for developmentally-oriented intervention strategies. In the absence of any specific predictions regarding the effects of high-level and low-level interactions it becomes difficult to demonstrate precise causal relations. The only demonstration of effectiveness of such an approach would be to verify what is self-evident —

that children placed in a wider more sensitive and responsive environment tend to make more rapid progress over a range of language and communication skills, compared to children in less stimulating environments. The precise speed and direction of the changes which occur will (and indeed must, as a precondition of language development), remain as much a function of the characteristics of the individual as to the specific experiences to which the child is exposed.

The problem for the language clinician is thus not simply one of playing a better game within the established rules. Instead, it is the more difficult problem of persuading the other players of the need to change the rules. It is necessary to persuade those professionals concerned with language therapy to abandon an outdated experimental methodology which, when translated into language intervention, inevitably becomes dominated by a concern for the prediction of specified outcomes in relation to variations in teaching input. Secondly, and at another level, it is necessary to reassure teachers that the best interests of language-disordered children are not always served by rigid timetabling, clear curriculum objectives and the overt demonstrations of didactic methods.

In the case of language development, it seems that children are likely to make most progress in relaxed play settings with peers or with child-centred adults. In this case a child-centred adult is one who is prepared to become involved in joint activities with the child, who is interested in understanding the child's intention and who is capable of responding in such a way that the child becomes aware of this understanding and at the same time is provided with opportunities for understanding the intentions of the adult. However, until a great deal more is known about the characteristics of natural social interactions between language-disordered children and their caretakers, it seems unlikely that any more detailed recommendations for intervention will be forthcoming.

In this chapter it has been argued that teaching and traditional forms of language intervention are incompatible with the *development* of *natural language* abilities in language-disordered children. It is suggested that instead of asking how to teach a pre-specified set of objectives, those concerned with language intervention should focus on *facilitating* development and then document retrospectively the emergence of each child's personal language curriculum.

Acknowledgements

I am indebted to Dr Graham Upton who provided valuable comments on an earlier draft of this paper and to Mrs E. Thomas who typed the manuscript.

References

Brinker, R.P. (1982) Contextual contours and the development of language, in M. Beveridge (ed.), *Children Thinking Through Language*, Edward Arnold, London

Chomsky, N. (1965) *Aspects of the Theory of Syntax* MIT Press, Cambridge, Mass.

Dunn, J., Wooding, C. and Hermann, J. (1977) Mothers speech to young children: variation in context, *Developmental Medicine and Child Neurology, 19*, 629-38

Francis, H. (1980) Language development and education, *Educational Analysis, 2*, 25-35

Fraser, C. and Roberts, N. (1975) Mothers' speech to children of four different ages, *Journal of Psycholinguistic Research, 4*, 9-17

Gillham, W.E.C. (1979) *The First Words Language Programme*, Allen & Unwin, London

——(1982) *Two Words Together*, Allen & Unwin, London

Harris, J. (1982) An ecological approach to facilitating linguistic interactions between severely mentally handicapped children and teachers in special schools, paper presented at the British Psychological Society Developmental Section Annual Conference, Durham, September, 1982

Hirst, P.H. (1973) What is teaching?, in R.S. Peters (ed.), *The Philosophy of Education*, Oxford University Press, Oxford

Leeming, K., Swann, W., Coupe, J. and Mittler, P. (1979) *Teaching Language and Communication to the Mentally Handicapped*, Schools Council Curriculum Bulletin No. 8., Evans/Methuen, London

Lock, A. (1980) Language development — past present and future, *Bulletin of the British Psychological Society, 33*, 5-8

MacDonald, J.D., Blott, J.P., Gordon, K., Spiegel, B. and Hartmann, M. (1974) An experimental parent-assisted treatment program for pre-school language delayed children, *Journal of Speech and Hearing Disorders, 31*, 395-415

Mahoney, G.J. (1975) Ethological approach to delayed language acquisition, *American Journal of Mental Deficiency, 80*, 139-48

——Crawley, S. and Pullis, M. (1980) Language intervention: models and issues, in B.K.Keogh (ed.), *Advances in Special Education Vol. 2*, JAl Press, Greenwich, Conn.

Miller, J.F. and Yoder, D.E. (1972) A syntax teaching program, in J.E. McLean, D.E. Yoder and R.L. Schiefelbusch (eds.), *Language Intervention and the Retarded: Developing Strategies*, University Park Press, Baltimore

——and Yoder, D.E. (1974) An ontegenetic language teaching strategy for retarded children, in R.L. Schiefelbusch and L.L. Lloyd (eds.), *Language Perspectives: Acquisition, Retardation and Intervention*, University Park Press, Baltimore

Muma, J.R. (1977) Language intervention strategies, *Language, Speech and Hearing Services in Schools, 8*, 107-25

Nelson, K. (1973) Structure and strategy in learning to talk, *Monographs of Society for Research in Child Development, 38*, 1-12, Serial No. 149
——(1980) Individual differences in language development: implications for development and language, *Developmental Psychology, 17*, 170-87

Newson, J. (1979) Intentional behaviour in the young infant, in H.R. Schaffer, and J. Dunn (eds.), *The First Year of Life*, John Wiley, Chichester

Rees, N.L. (1978) Pragmatics of language acquisition, in R.L. Schiefelbusch (ed.), *Bases of Language Intervention*, Park Press, Baltimore

Ruder, N. (1978) Planning and programming for language intervention, in R.L. Schiefelbusch (ed.), *Bases of Language Intervention*, University Park Press, Baltimore

Ryan, J. (1973) Interpretation and imitation in early language development, in R.A. Hinde and I. Stevenson-Hinde (eds.), *Constraints on Learning: Limitation and Predispositions*, Academic Press, London

Sameroff, A. (1975) Transactional models in early social relations, *Human Development, 18*, 65-79

Seibert, J.M. and Kimbrough Oller, D. (1981) Linguistic pragmatics and language intervention strategies, *Journal of Autism and Developmental Disorders, 11*, 1

Seitz, S. (1975) Language intervention: changing the language environment of the retarded child, in R. Koch and F. De La Cruz (eds.), *Down's Syndrome (Mongolism) Research, Prevention and Management*, Brunner/Mazel Inc., New York

Shotter, J. (1982) Models of childhood in British developmental research, invited paper at the British Psychological Society Developmental Section Annual Conference, Durham, September

Skinner, B.F. (1957) *Verbal Behavior*, Appleton-Century Crofts, New York

Tizard, B., Hughes, M., Carmichael, H. and Pinkerton, G. (1983) Children's questions and adults answers, *Journal of Child Psychology and Psychiatry, 24*, 269-82

Wood, D.J., MacMahon, L. and Cranstoun, Y. (1980) *Working with Under-Fives*, Grant McIntyre, London

CONTRIBUTORS

DEREK BLACKMAN is Professor and Head of the Department of Psychology at University College, Cardiff, He was President of the British Psychological Society in 1981/2, and is currently editor of the *British Journal of Psychology*. His principal interests are contemporary behaviourism, especially operant conditioning, and psychopharmacology. He is the author of *Operant Conditioning* (Methuen, 1974), and co-editor with D.J. Sanger of *Contemporary Research in Behavioral Pharmacology* (Plenum, 1978) and *Aspects of Psychopharmacology* (Methuen, 1984), and with D.J. Müller and A.J. Chapman of *Psychology and Law. Topics From an International Conference* (Wiley, 1984).

GILLIAN CLEZY is a practising Speech Pathologist and Lecturer in Therapeutic Processes and Aural Rehabilitation at the School of Communication Disorders at the Lincoln Institute of Health Sciences, Melbourne, Australia. She was trained in the United Kingdom and initially worked at the Audiology Research Unit in Reading, Berkshire. Much of her twenty years of clinical experience has been in general hospitals, in both England and Australia. She has always maintained an interest in profound hearing loss and mother/child interaction and carried out the first infant screening programme to detect deafness in an Australian population. She has just completed a longitudinal linguistic study into the effects of conductive hearing loss on both members of the mother/child dyad.

ENA DAVIES is currently Senior Lecturer in Speech Pathology at the South Glamorgan Institute of Higher Education, Cardiff. Prior to this appointment she was Chief Speech Therapist at the University Hospital of Wales, Cardiff. Having worked for the Spastics Society for twelve years her major clinical experience has been with cerebral palsied children and adults. She is Advisor on Cerebral Palsy to the College of Speech Therapists and is the UK Advisor on Blissymbolics Communication.

JOHN HARRIS was awarded a B.A. in Psychology at University College, Swansea, in 1973 and then moved to the Child Development Research Unit at Nottingham University where he studied for an M.A.

243

in Child Development and subsequently a Ph.D. After lecturing in the Department of Education, Trent Polytechnic, he returned to Wales where he is currently lecturer in child development in the Department of Education, University College, Cardiff.

PATRICIA HOWLIN is Senior Lecturer in the Departments of Psychology and Child and Adolescent Psychiatry at the Institute of Psychiatry, London, and Honorary Principal Psychologist in the Children's Department at the Maudsley Hospital. Her clinical work is concerned with the treatment of autistic individuals at home and in the community and this is one of her main areas of research. Another of her interests is work on language development.

ANITA JOHNSON took her M.S. from the University of Arizona in 1970. She was a research associate at the University of Arizona from 1970 through 1979. Subsequently she has served as a public school speech-language pathologist.

CHRIS KIERNAN is Deputy Director of the Thomas Coram Research Unit. He has been involved in research with severely mentally handicapped children and young people since 1970. His main interest is in the investigation of factors affecting behavioural change and, in particular, in the translation of research findings into practice. He will become Director of the Hester Adrian Research Centre, University of Manchester, in 1984.

ROY McCONKEY is Senior Research Officer with St. Michael's House, a Dublin-based organisation providing services to mentally handicapped people and their families. He is also part-time lecturer in the Department of Remedial Linguistics, Trinity College, Dublin. His particular research interests are play and language intervention, parental involvement and community education about disability. He is co-author of several books, giving practical advice to parents and staff – *Let Me Speak, Let Me Play, Let's Make Toys* (Souvenir Press) and he has published articles in many professional journals.

JAMES McLEAN is Senior Scientist, Bureau of Child Research, University of Kansas, and Director of the Parsons Research Center, Parsons, Kansas. He also holds appointments as Courtesy Professor in the Department of Speech, Language, Hearing: Sciences and Disorders and the Department of Human Development and Family Life at

Kansas. Prior to his current appointments at Kansas, he was Professor of Special Education and Chairman of the Department at George Peabody College for Teachers. He received the B.S. degree in speech pathology from Indiana University in 1951; the M.A. degree in speech pathology from the University of Kansas in 1959; and the Ph.D. degree in speech pathology and audiology from the University of Kansas in 1965.

DONALD MOWRER received his Master of Science degree in 1953 from Florida State University and a Doctorate of Philosophy from Arizona State University in 1964. He has been professor in the Department of Speech and Hearing Science at Arizona State University since 1965. His chief interest is in the application of the principles of behaviour therapy to the remediation of communication disorders. He has written several books, chapters, and numerous articles about this topic. He has lectured in many foreign countries including a semester lectureship in 1982 at the University of Cape Town, South Africa. He is a Fellow in the American Speech and Hearing Association.

DAVE MÜLLER is Senior Lecturer in the School of Psychology at Preston Polytechnic. His research interests are in applied social and cognitive psychology. He has written and edited five books, including (with C. Code, eds) *Aphasia Therapy* (Edward Arnold, London, 1983) and (with C. Code and S. Munro) *Language Assessment for Remediation* (Croom Helm, London, 1981). Currently he is associate and review editor of the *British Journal of Psychology*.

RALPH SHELTON took his Ph.D. from the University of Utah in 1959. From 1959 through 1970 he was a professor in the Hearing and Speech Department of the University of Kansas School of Medicine. Subsequently he has been Professor of Speech and Hearing Science at the University of Arizona. Much of his research has been supported by the National Institute of Dental Research, Department of Health and Human Services, United States Public Health Service. He is former editor of the *Journal of Speech and Hearing Disorders* and past-president of the American Cleft Palate Association.

LEE K. SNYDER-MCLEAN is a Research Associate with the Bureau of Child Research, University of Kansas. She also holds courtesy appointments as Assistant Professor with the Departments of Human Development and Family Life, Special Education and Speech,

Language, Hearing: Sciences and Disorders. She has worked as a classroom teacher of the mentally retarded and most recently has directed a model early intervention programme for handicapped infants and young children. McLean received her B.S. degree from Syracuse University, her M.Ed. from the University of Washington and her Ph.D. from George Peabody College for Teachers.

AUTHOR INDEX

Addison, R.M. 26, 50
Adelson, E. 117, 132
Allen, D. 200, 224
Allen, E. 230
Andersen, E.S. 65, 78, 81
Anderson, C.A. 51
Anderson, L. 202, 228
Apolloni, T. 203, 228
Armfield, A. 183, 188, 196
Arndt, W.B. 32, 54, 148, 149, 156, 201, 229
Attwood, T. 206, 208, 223
Augustine, L.E. 201, 204, 210, 213, 224
Aulman-Rupp, A. 98, 112
Ayllon, T. 27, 50
Azrin, N.H. 27, 50

Baer, D.M. 25, 30, 42, 50, 52, 54, 63, 81, 120, 132, 175, 188, 189, 190-2, 195, 196, 205, 225, 228-9
Bailey, R.D. 186-7, 194
Baird, V.G. 143, 155
Baker, B. 221, 224
Baker, R.L. 36, 53, 145, 155
Bakker-Rennes, H. 98, 110
Bandura, A. 46, 50
Bannon, J.B. 37, 50
Bar-Adon, A. 55, 81
Barnes, R. 195, 196
Barnes, S. 198-9, 223
Bartak, L. 117, 119, 133
Bates, E. 43, 48, 51, 55, 58-62, 64, 66, 72-3, 78, 81, 129, 131, 176-7, 194
Bax, M. 201, 229
Bell, R.Q. 142, 156
Benedict, H. 198, 224
Benigni, L. 61, 81
Bennett, C.W. 201, 203, 207. 210, 223
Bercovici, N. 197, 225
Bereiter, C. 34-5, 49, 51
Berger, M. 197, 201, 206, 218, 225-6, 228, 230
Berkovitz, B.P. 197, 205, 223, 229
Bernstein, B. 33, 51

Beveridge, M. 241
Bicknell, D.J. 187, 194
Bidder, R. 202, 223-4
Bijou, S.W. 25, 51, 197, 225
Birnbraver, J.S. 26, 29, 51
Blackman, D.E. 1, 6, 17, 189
Blackwell, J. 200, 224
Blackwell, L. 213, 225
Bloch, J. 202, 211, 223
Bloom, L. 45, 49, 52, 71-2, 79, 81, 87, 100, 110, 136, 154, 184, 196
Blott, J.P. 201, 223, 227, 231, 241
Blunden, R. 202, 228
Boone, D.R. 87, 94, 110
Bornstein, H. 182, 195
Bosler, S. 141, 147, 154
Bower, G.H. 14
Bowerman, M.F. 72, 79, 81
Bowser, D.C. 141-2, 156
Bradfield, R.H. 51-2, 54
Branston, M. 124, 133
Brasel, K. 211, 214, 223
Bretherton, I. 61, 81
Bricker, D.D. 131, 197, 225
Bricker, W.A. 175, 194
Brinker, R.P. 239, 241
Brodbeck, A.J. 33, 51
Broen, P.D. 136, 154
Brookshire, R.H. 32, 51
Brose, D. 229
Brown, F. 33, 51
Brown, I. 89, 111
Brown, L. 195-6
Brown, Roger 77, 81, 88, 92-3, 100, 110, 198-9, 223
Brown, R. 197, 201-2, 209, 226
Bruner, J. 43-4, 49, 51, 61-2, 69, 71, 75, 77, 81, 100, 110, 119, 131, 176, 194
Bryant, G. 202, 223-4
Bryen, D.N. 225
Buckholdt, D. 213, 225
Buckley, M.K. 48, 54
Buell, J. 229
Buium, N. 200, 223
Bullock, A. 138, 154
Burchard, J.D. 26, 29, 51

247

SUBJECT INDEX